Applications of Neural Networks in Environment, Energy, and Health

Progress in Neural Processing • 5

Applications of Neural Networks in Environment, Energy, and Health

Proceedings of the 1995 Workshop on Environmental and Energy Applications of Neural Networks

Richland, Washington, USA 30–31 March 1995

Editors

Paul E. Keller
Pacific Northwest National Laboratory, USA

Sherif Hashem
Cairo University, Egypt

Lars J. Kangas
Pacific Northwest National Laboratory, USA

Richard T. Kouzes
West Virginia University, USA

World Scientific
Singapore • New Jersey • London • Hong Kong

Published by

World Scientific Publishing Co. Pte. Ltd.

P O Box 128, Farrer Road, Singapore 912805

USA office: Suite 1B, 1060 Main Street, River Edge, NJ 07661

UK office: 57 Shelton Street, Covent Garden, London WC2H 9HE

Library of Congress Cataloging-in-Publication Data

Workshop on Environmental and Energy Applications of Neural Networks (1995 : Richland, Wash.)

Applications of neural networks in environment, energy, and health ; proceedings of the 1995 Workshop on Environmental and Energy Applications of Neural Networks, Pacific Northwest National Laboratory, Richland, Washington, USA, 30–31 March 1995 / edited by Paul E. Keller,

p. cm. -- (Progress in neural processing)

Includes bibliographical references.

ISBN 9810227582

1. Neural networks (Computer science) -- Congresses. 2. Environmental protection -- Data processing -- Congresses. 3. Power resources -- Data processing -- Congresses. 4. Medical sciences -- Data processing -- Congresses. I. Keller, Paul E. II. Title. III. Series.

QA76.87.W675 1995

620'.00285'63--dc20 96-20283

CIP

British Library Cataloguing-in-Publication Data

A catalogue record for this book is available from the British Library.

Printed in Singapore.

CONTENTS

Sponsors

The *Workshop on Environmental and Energy Applications of Neural Networks* was sponsored by the Environmental Molecular Sciences Laboratory, Energy Technology Development Initiative, Medical Technology and Systems Initiative, and Applied Physics Center at Pacific Northwest National Laboratory; and by the Richland Section of the Institute of Electrical and Electronics Engineers.

Pacific Northwest National Laboratory

Pacific Northwest National Laboratory is a multiprogram national laboratory operated for the U.S. Department of Energy by Battelle Memorial Institute under contract DE-AC06-76RLO 1830.

Pacific Northwest National Laboratory's core mission is to deliver environmental science and technology in the service of the nation and humanity. Through basic research we create fundamental knowledge of natural, engineered, and social systems that is the basis for both effective environmental technology and sound public policy. We solve legacy environmental problems by delivering technologies that remediate existing environmental hazards, addressing today's environmental needs with technologies that prevent pollution and minimize waste, and are laying the technical foundation for tomorrow's inherently clean energy and industrial processes. We also apply our capabilities to meet selected national security, energy, and human health needs, to strengthen the U.S. economy, and to support the education of future scientists and engineers.

Pacific Northwest National Laboratory acts as a steward of the U.S. Department of Energy's resources by anticipating future national needs and investing in the development of major new capabilities and programs to meet these needs. Current investments include molecular science research, advanced processing technology, biotechnology, global environmental change research and energy technology development.

Preface

This book contains edited versions of the technical presentations made at the *Workshop on Environmental and Energy Applications of Neural Networks (WEEANN '95). WEEANN '95* was held on 30-31 March 1995 at Pacific Northwest National Laboratory in Richland, Washington, USA. The workshop attracted researchers and practitioners from the USA, Canada, and Russia. Participants represented U.S. Department of Energy national laboratories (Idaho National Engineering Laboratory, Pacific Northwest National Laboratory, and Sandia National Laboratories), U.S. Department of Energy site contractors (ICF Kaiser and Westinghouse Hanford Company), U.S. Bureau of Reclamation, academia (Colorado School of Mines, Moscow State University, New York Medical College, Rollins College, Technical University of Nova Scotia, Tennessee State University, Texas A&M University, University of Alberta, University of Idaho, University of Maryland, University of Washington, Washington State University, and Western Washington University), industry (BH Engineering Systems Limited, Chelan County Public Utility District, Computer Science Innovations, Dendronic Decisions Limited, Honeywell Technology Center, Perkin-Elmer Corporation, Siemens Corporate Research, Stirling Technology Company, and Westinghouse), and research institutes (Battelle Memorial Institute, British Columbia Cancer Agency, and Electric Power Research Institute).

The purpose of the workshop was to provide a forum for discussing environmental, energy, and biomedical applications of neural networks. Panels were held to discuss research and development issues relating to real-world applications in each of the three areas. The applications covered in the workshop were:

- **Environmental Applications:** Modeling and predicting soil, air and water pollution; waste reduction; environmental sensing; spectroscopy; hazardous waste handling and cleanup; and environmental monitoring for power systems.
- **Energy Applications:** Process monitoring and optimization of power systems, modeling and control of power plants, environmental monitoring for power systems, power load forecasting, and fault location and diagnosis of power systems.
- **Biomedical/Health Applications:** Medical image and signal analysis, medical diagnosis, analysis of environmental health effects, health insurance, and modeling biological systems.

In Chapter 1, Tariq Samad from Honeywell Technology Center discusses his insights into the practical application of neural networks to environmental and energy technologies. In Chapter 2, Radu Drossu and Zoran Obradović from Washington

State University discuss the relationship between stochastic models and neural network approaches to time series modeling.

Chapters 3 through 10 cover environmental applications of neural networks. Many of these applications involve U.S. Department of Energy (DOE) laboratories and sites. In Chapter 3, Manavendra Misra and his colleagues from Colorado School of Mines summarize their work in interpreting electromagnetic and magnetic sensor information with neural networks for the DOE's Idaho National Engineering Laboratory. In Chapter 4, Paul E. Keller and his colleagues at the DOE's Pacific Northwest National Laboratory and the DOE's Hanford Site discuss the application of neural networks to the analysis of nuclear spectra for use in isotope identification and waste handling. In Chapter 5, Greg Becker from the DOE's Idaho National Engineering Laboratory discusses initial investigations of neural networks in nondestructive transuranic waste assay. In Chapter 6, Tomas Lopez and Barbara L. Philipp from the DOE's Hanford Site along with a colleague from Washington State University discuss the application of neural networks to determine moisture content in humidity-attenuated near infrared spectra. In Chapter 7, Yuri V. Orlov and his colleagues at Moscow State University and the Institute of Ecology discuss a neural network approach to fluorescent diagnostics of organic pollution in natural waters. In Chapter 8, David G. Robinson of the DOE's Sandia National Laboratories discusses the applications of neural networks to reliability and risk analysis. In Chapter 9, Sherif Hashem and his colleagues at the DOE's Pacific Northwest National Laboratory discuss electronic noses and their applications to environmental sensing. In Chapter 10, Ferial El-Hawary from BH Engineering Systems Limited discusses neural network based prediction of atmospheric pollutant concentrations from fossil-fired power plant emissions.

Chapters 11 through 16 cover energy applications of neural networks. Most of these applications deal with electrical power delivery or electrical component reliability. In Chapter 11, Dejan J. Sobajic from the Electric Power Research Institute discusses neural network control strategies to improve power system performance. In Chapter 12, William W. Armstrong and his colleagues at Dendronic Decisions Limited and the University of Alberta discuss adaptive logic networks and their ability to predict compressor unit failure. In Chapter 13, Monte F. Hancock from Computer Science Innovations discusses near and long-term load prediction with radial bases function neural networks. In Chapter 14, Rex C. Stratton and Krista L. Gaustad from the DOE's Pacific Northwest National Laboratory discuss a neural network approach to distribution short-term load forecasting. In Chapter 15, Robert J. Streifel, Robert J. Marks, and their colleagues at the University of Washington propose a neural network based method to monitor, detect and localize shorts in power system devices. In Chapter 16, Satinderpaul S. Devgan and Dusty R.

Walker, Jr. from Tennessee State University discuss neural network based wind prediction for a hybrid wind power storage and generation system.

Chapters 17 through 24 cover neural network applications in medicine and health care. In Chapter 17, Harry B. Burke from New York Medical College discusses the importance of artificial neural networks in biomedicine. In Chapter 18, William W. Armstrong and his colleagues at Dendronic Decisions Limited and the University of Alberta discuss adaptive logic networks and their application in rehabilitation of persons with incomplete spinal cord injury. In Chapter 19, Raymond Watrous and his colleagues at Siemens Corporate Research discuss the application of neural network tools to electro-cardiogram patient monitoring. In Chapter 20, Yuri V. Orlov and his colleagues at Moscow State University discuss a neural network based diagnostic system for the detection and analysis of auditory evoked potentials. In Chapter 21, David D. Turner from the DOE's Pacific Northwest National Laboratory and Edwin R. Holmes from Sacred Heart Medical Center discuss the diagnosis of coronary artery disease with a backpropagation neural network. In Chapter 22, Thomas LoFaro from Washington State University and Nancy Kopell from Boston University discuss a model of the dynamics of a network of coupled biological neurons. In Chapter 23, Monte F. Hancock from Computer Science Innovations discusses estimation of workman's compensation claims with radial bases function neural networks. In Chapter 24, Lars J. Kangas and his colleagues at the DOE's Pacific Northwest National Laboratory and Life Link Incorporated discuss a novel approach to modeling and diagnosing the cardiovascular system with neural networks.

Workshop Organizing Committee

Sherif Hashem (Chairman)	shashem@ritsec.com.eg	+20 (2) 349-6055
Paul E. Keller (Editor)	pe_keller@pnl.gov	+1 (509) 375-2254
Lars J. Kangas	lj_kangas@pnl.gov	+1 (509) 375-3905
Richard T. Kouzes	rkouzes@wvnvm.wvnet.edu	+1 (304) 293-6667
Rex (Trav) C. Statton	rc_stratton@pnl.gov	+1 (509) 375-2779
Janice K.Gunter	jk_gunter@pnl.gov	+1 (509) 375-2350

Mailing Address:

Pacific Northwest National Laboratory
P.O. Box 999, MS K1-87
Richland, Washington 99352, USA
Facsimile: +1 (509) 375-6631

Acknowledgments

The workshop organizers wish to again thank the workshop Keynote speakers: Gerald L. Work (Associate Laboratory Director), Bernard F. Saffell (Energy Technology Development Initiative program manager), and Barbara A. Fecht (Medical Technology and Systems Initiative program manager). We also thank the authors and panelists for excellent presentations and insightful discussions. Further, we express our appreciation for the support and assistance of the staff of the Pacific Northwest National Laboratory, with our most sincere thanks to Janice Gunter, Pamela Stanley, Cary Counts, Jan Lewis, Rex (Trav) Stratton, Krista Gaustad, and Richard May.

Additional Information

Additional information about the workshop and neural network related research at the Pacific Northwest National Laboratory may be obtained from the World Wide Web at:

`http://www.emsl.pnl.gov:2080/docs/cie/neural/workshop2/`

WEEANN '95 Program

WEDNESDAY, MARCH 29, 1995

6:00 p.m. – 7:00 p.m.	Registration.
6:30 p.m. – 9:30 p.m.	Introduction to Neural Networks (Tutorial). *P.E. Keller, L.J. Kangas, and S. Hashem.*

THURSDAY, MARCH 30, 1995

7:30 a.m. – 8:30 a.m.	Registration.

OPENING SESSION *(chair: S. Hashem)*

8:00 a.m. – 8:05 a.m.	Workshop Opening. *R.T. Kouzes and S. Hashem.*
8:05 a.m. – 8:25 a.m.	Overview of the Pacific Northwest National Laboratory. *G.L. Work.*
8:25 a.m. – 9:05 a.m.	Neural Network Models: Insights and Prescriptions from Practical Applications (invited talk). *T. Samad. Honeywell Technology Center, Minneapolis, Minnesota, USA.*
9:05 a.m. – 9:45 a.m.	Application of Computational Neural Networks in Predicting Atmospheric Pollutant Concentrations due to Fossil-fired Electric Power Generation (invited talk). *F. El-Hawary. BH Engineering Systems Ltd. & Technical University of Nova Scotia, Halifax, Nova Scotia, Canada.*
9:45 a.m. – 10:25 a.m.	Neural Network Analysis for Hazardous Waste Characterization (invited talk). *M. Misra, L.Y. Pratt, C. Farris, and R.O. Hansen. Colorado School of Mines, Golden, Colorado, USA.*
10:25 a.m. – 10:40 a.m.	Break.

ENVIRONMENTAL SESSION *(chair: P.E. Keller)*

10:40 a.m. – 10:50 a.m.	Overview of the Environmental Molecular Sciences Laboratory. *R.T. Kouzes.*
10:50 a.m. – 11:10 a.m.	Neural Networks for Nuclear Spectroscopy. *P.E. Keller, L.J. Kangas, S. Hashem, and R.T. Kouzes, Pacific Northwest National Laboratory, and G.L. Troyer, Westinghouse Hanford Company, Richland, Washington, USA.*
11:10 a.m. – 11:30 a.m.	A Hybrid Neural Network Structure for Application to Nondestructive Transuranic Waste Assay. *G. Becker.*

	Idaho National Engineering Laboratory, Idaho Falls, Idaho, USA.
11:30 a.m. – 11:50 a.m.	Application of Neural Networks to Determine Moisture Content on Humidity-Attenuated Near Infrared Spectra. *T. Lopez, Westinghouse Hanford Company, Richland, Washington, USA; B.L. Philipp, ICF Kaiser, Richland, Washington, USA; and Thompson-Bachmeier, Washington State University, Pullman, Washington, USA.*
11:50 a.m. – 12:10 p.m.	Fluorescent Diagnostics of Organic Pollution in Natural Waters: A Neural Network Approach. *Yu.V. Orlov, I.G. Persiantsev, and S.P. Rebrik, Moscow State University, Moscow, Russia; and S.M. Babichenko, Institute of Ecology, Tallinn, Estonia.*
12:10 p.m. – 1:00 p.m.	Lunch.
1:00 p.m. – 1:20 p.m.	Reliability and Risk Analysis Using Artificial Neural Networks. *D. Robinson. Sandia National Laboratories, Albuquerque, New Mexico, USA.*
1:20 p.m. – 1:40 p.m.	Electronic Noses and Their Applications in Environmental Monitoring. *S. Hashem, P.E. Keller, R.T. Kouzes, and L.J. Kangas. Pacific Northwest National Laboratory, Richland, Washington, USA.*
1:40 p.m. – 2:30 p.m.	Panel Discussion on Environmental Applications. *S. Hashem, F. El-Hawary, M. Misra, and G.L. Troyer*
2:30 p.m. – 2:45 p.m.	Break.

ENERGY SESSION *(chairs: R.C. Stratton, K.L. Gaustad, and S. Hashem)*

2:45 p.m. – 3:00 p.m.	Introduction and Overview of the Energy Technology Development Initiative. *B.F. Saffell*
3:00 p.m. – 3:40 p.m.	Investigation of Neural-Net Based Control Strategies for Improved Power System Dynamic Performance (invited talk). *D. Sobajic. Electric Power Research Institute, Palo Alto, California, USA.*
3:40 p.m. – 4:00 p.m.	Feasibility of using Adaptive Logic Networks to Predict Compressor Unit Failure. *W.W. Armstrong, C. Chu, and M.M. Thomas. Dendronic Decisions Ltd., Edmonton, Alberta, Canada.*
4:00 p.m. – 4:20 p.m.	Stochastic Modeling Hints for Neural Network Prediction. *R. Drossu and Z. Obradović. Washington State University, Pullman, Washington, USA.*

4:20 p.m. – 4:40 p.m.	Near and Long-Term Load Prediction Using Radial Basis Function Networks. *M.F. Hancock. Computer Science Innovations Corporation (Melbourne, Florida) & Rollins College (Winter Park, Florida), USA.*
4:40 p.m. – 5:00 p.m.	An Approach to Distribution Short-Term Load Forecasting. *R.C. Stratton and K.L. Gaustad, Pacific Northwest National Laboratory, Richland, Washington, USA.*
5:00 p.m. – 6:00 p.m.	Break.
6:00 p.m. – 9:00 p.m.	Dinner at the Best Western–Tower Inn.

FRIDAY, MARCH 31, 1995

8:00 a.m. – 8:10 a.m.	Workshop announcements.
8:10 a.m. – 8:50 a.m.	Twin Signal Signature Sensing: Application to Shorted Winding Monitoring, Detection and Localization (invited talk). *R.J. Marks II, M.A. El-Sharkawi, R.J. Streifel, and I. Kerszenbaum. University of Washington, Seattle, Washington, USA.*
8:50 a.m. – 9:10 a.m.	Design of a Hybrid Wind Power Storage and Generation System for a Remote Community. *S.S. Devgan and D.R. Walker, Jr. Tennessee State University, Nashville, Tennessee, USA.*
9:10 a.m. – 10:20 a.m.	Panel Discussion on Energy Applications. *R.C. Stratton, B.F. Saffell, T. Samad, W.W. Armstrong, D.J. Sobajic*
10:20 a.m. – 10:40 a.m.	Break.

BIOMEDICAL SESSION *(chairs: L.J. Kangas and P.E. Keller)*

10:40 a.m. – 10:50 a.m.	Introduction and overview of the Medical Technologies and Systems Initiative. *B.A. Fecht .*
10:50 a.m. – 11:30 a.m.	The Importance of Artificial Neural Networks in Biomedicine (invited talk). *H.B. Burke. New York Medical College, Valhalla, New York, USA.*
11:30 a.m. – 12:10 p.m.	Adaptive Logic Networks in Rehabilitation (invited talk). *W.W. Armstrong, A. Kostov, R.B. Stein, and M.M. Thomas. Dendronic Decisions Ltd., Edmonton, Alberta, Canada.*
12:10 p.m. – 1:00 p.m.	Lunch.
1:00 p.m. – 1:40 p.m.	Synthesize, Optimize, Analyze, Repeat (SOAR): Application Of Neural Network Tools To ECG Patient Monitoring (invited talk). *R.L. Watrous, G. Towell, and*

	M.S. Glassman. Siemens Corporate Research, Princeton, New Jersey, USA.
1:40 p.m. – 2:00 p.m.	Diagnostic System for Detection and Analysis of Auditory Evoked Potentials. *Yu.V. Orlov, I.G. Persiantsev, S.P. Rebrik, A.A. Deviatov, Ju.S. Shugai, and A.V. Kurganskij. Moscow State University, Moscow, Russia.*
2:00 p.m. – 2:20 p.m.	Diagnosing Coronary Artery Disease with a Backpropagation Neural Network: Lessons Learned. *D.D. Turner, Pacific Northwest National Laboratory, Richland, Washington, USA; and E.R. Holmes, III, Sacred Heart Medical Center, Spokane, Washington, USA.*
2:20 p.m. – 2:40 p.m.	Reduction of a Network of Voltage Gated Conductance Equations to a One-Dimensional Map. *T. LoFaro. Washington State University, Pullman, Washington, USA; and Nancy Koppel, Boston University, Boston, Massachusetts, USA.*
2:40 p.m. – 3:00 p.m.	Estimating Dollar-Value Outcomes of Workman's Compensation Claims Using Radial Basis Function Networks. *M.F. Hancock. Computer Science Innovations Corporation (Melbourne, Florida) & Rollins College (Winter Park, Florida), USA.*
3:00 p.m. – 3:20 p.m.	Break.
3:20 p.m. – 3:40 p.m.	Cardiovascular Modeling and Diagnostics. *L.J. Kangas, P.E. Keller, S. Hashem, and R.T. Kouzes, Pacific Northwest National Laboratory, Richland, Washington, USA; and P.A. Allen, Life Link Incorporated, Richland, Washington, USA.*
3:40 p.m. – 4:30 p.m.	Panel Discussion on Biomedical Applications. *P.E. Keller, R.T. Kouzes, H.B. Burke, R.L. Watrous, and W.W. Armstrong*
4:30 p.m. – 5:00 p.m.	Wrap up and concluding remarks. *S. Hashem.*

1. NEURAL NETWORK MODELS: INSIGHTS AND PRESCRIPTIONS FROM PRACTICAL APPLICATIONS

TARIQ SAMAD
Honeywell Technology Center, 3660 Technology Drive
Minneapolis, Minnesota 55418, USA
E-mail: samad@htc.honeywell.com

1.1. Introduction

Neural networks appear to have successfully weathered the transition from research to practice. For many nonlinear modeling problems, they are now the technology of first choice, and numerous successes in industrial applications attest to their utility. In the course of developing these applications, practitioners have been faced with a variety of issues – issues that are often of secondary concern in research contexts. This paper briefly discusses several of these, noting in particular the rich connections between neural networks and other, conventional technologies.

For a variety of reasons, researchers and application developers from a broad variety of fields have been drawn to neural networks. The resulting interaction has been remarkably synergistic. Neural networks have become a popular modeling tool in these fields, and, at the same time, it has become apparent that a wealth of theory and methodology already exists that can help address numerous problems in practical applications of neural networks.

Our focus here is on neural networks as modeling technology. However, much of the discussion is also relevant to other types of applications such as classification, control, and optimization.

1.2. Some Important Aspects of Neural Network Applications

1.2.1. Generalization

Neural networks – at least the conventional ones that are currently in vogue for modeling applications – are essentially nonparametric regression models. Nonparametric modeling is the term used in statistics for "black-box" or model-free estimation, where a large number of parameters are used and few structural assumptions are made about the model. A well-known difficulty with nonparametric models is that they have a tendency to overfit. The large number of parameters provide a degree of modeling flexibility that the available data may not warrant.

Much has been written about neural networks and overfits. The whole enterprise of neural network modeling as we know it has been questioned as untenable (Poggio and Girosi 1990; Geman, Bienenstock, and Geman 1992). On the other hand, innumerable applications attest to the fact that models with excellent generalization properties can be developed if care is exercised.

A resolution of this paradoxical situation has been suggested by Sjöberg and Ljung (1992): the use of a test set to terminate training before complete convergence on the training set is attained. It turns out that early termination of an iterative model development algorithm is closely related to "regularization", which is a well-known approach in statistics for overcoming the overfitting tendency of nonparametric regressions. Regularization ensures that the model satisfies some smoothness constraints and, in a quantifiable sense, so does early termination. Smoothness is realized in both cases through a reduction in the number of effective model parameters.

The use of a test set in the termination criterion implies that performance on the test set is not an accurate measure of model accuracy. A third data set, sometimes referred to as "validation" data, is recommended in such cases. The validation set is only used to assess the goodness of the model after its development is complete. This approach may not be feasible if data is limited, and alternatives such as cross validation schemes are a recourse.

Another approach to achieving good generalization is to reduce the number of actual model parameters. Network pruning algorithms have been developed for this purpose that, during training, excise weights that are analyzed as not necessary (e.g., Le Cun, Denker, and Solla 1990). Although these algorithms are often complicated, pruning may eventually provide a generic solution to the generalization problem.

1.2.2. Learning or Optimization.

The subject of supervised learning for neural networks has generated a mini-industry, and generating a backpropagation improvement is almost an initiation rite for neural neophytes. We often think of "learning" as a distinctive aspect of neural network technology, and of learning algorithms such as "backpropagation" as major novel contributions. In fact, neural network supervised learning is a nonlinear optimization problem (and a relatively simple one in that no constraints are involved).

Once the learning = optimization equation is recognized, learning algorithms can be related to well-known methods in the optimization literature. Vanilla backpropagation is an approximate version of gradient descent – the fidelity of the approximation depends, for example, on whether weight updates are interleaved with gradient computation or not, whether epoch updating or pattern updating is in effect, and on the step size. Analogously, backpropagation with momentum is an approximate version of conjugate gradient (Leonard and Kramer 1990).

One may well ask why we need to resort to approximations. In fact, true conjugate gradient (e.g., Fletcher and Reeves 1964) seems to be gaining increasing popularity as the learning algorithm of choice for practical applications. Compared to backpropagation with momentum, conjugate gradient converges faster and does not require the manual specification of learning and momentum rates. Good results have also been reported in small-to-moderate-size applications with another nonlinear optimization algorithm, the quasi-Newton Levenberg-Marquardt (Marquardt 1963).

It is worth remarking that approximations can sometimes outperform the real item. There is considerable anecdotal evidence that backpropagation will converge more reliably (although much less rapidly) than true gradient descent or true conjugate gradient. The occasional uphill moves that result from the approximations can be effective in escaping local minima, it seems.

A fundamental distinction in nonlinear optimization is that between gradient-based and non-gradient-based algorithms. The algorithms mentioned above are in the former category. Nongradient-based algorithms, in particular evolutionary computing methods, are attracting considerable interest and may be practicable in the foreseeable future. Their primary attractions are a reduced likelihood of converging to a poor local minimum and a capability to tolerate nonstandard, and nondifferentiable, optimization criteria. Thus criteria of practical interest can be used directly instead of first transforming them into a suitable analytic form (e.g., quadratic).

1.2.3. Algebraic Versus Dynamic Models

Neural network models such as the multilayer perceptron are algebraic structures – they have no state or memory. Hence the output of a given network at any time depends purely on its current inputs. In many applications, however, we are interested in capturing the transient behavior of real systems – i.e., in developing dynamic models. Modeling dynamics requires that history be taken into account. The common approach is to include appropriate dynamic information as network input. Thus, in addition to the current value of system input, the network may be given some number of past values of system inputs and outputs. This is a nonlinear extension of a linear ARMA-like (Auto-Regressive Moving Average) model widely used in system identification.

With input/output data from a system, a neural network dynamic model can be developed in straightforward fashion using conventional supervised learning (e.g., backpropagation or conjugate gradient). During the training process, actual inputs and outputs from the system are provided as network inputs and the target output is the value of the system output at the next time step. The network is trained as a one-step-ahead predictor. For longer term predictions, model outputs from previous time steps must be used as input in place of actual process outputs. Unfortunately, model accuracy can degrade rather quickly as longer-term predictions are attempted, especially if limited data is available for training and it is corrupted with realistic noise levels.

Neural network models that are more accurate long-term predictors can be developed if model outputs are used during learning instead of actual process outputs (Su, McAvoy, and Werbos 1992). This "externally recurrent" network design severely complicates the learning algorithm, since conventional supervised learning is no longer possible (the collected data no longer includes all the network inputs, some of which are now neural network outputs from prior time steps). The key issue is the computation of gradients of the cost function (modeling error) with respect to the model parameters (neural network weights). For dynamical systems such as externally recurrent networks, an efficient algorithm for gradient computation is "backpropagation through time" (Werbos 1990). This is equivalent to a calculus of variations method, also known as the adjoint method (Bryson and Ho 1975). Su *et. al.* (1992) demonstrate dramatic improvements in accuracy of long-term prediction for two industrial processes: wastewater treatment and catalytic reforming.

The distinction between these two types of dynamic model development approaches is well-known in system identification. The approaches are often referred to as equation error identification (for the case where process output is used for model input) and output error identification (for the case where model output is fed back as model input). For linear dynamic models, equation error identification is a linear algebra exercise that can be solved with a matrix pseudo-inversion whereas output error identification requires an iterative algorithm.

Finally, we note that dynamic neural networks – neural network architectures that have state or memory typically implemented through internal feedback connections – can be used for developing dynamic models. In this case, dynamic information need not be provided as external input. Again, backpropagation through time is needed for learning. Dynamic neural networks are an exciting research topic, and recently developed Kalman-filter-based estimation methods promise practical benefits in the near future (Puskorius and Feldkamp 1994).

1.2.4. Input Selection.

In the synthetic problems that are the (justified) recourse for testing new modeling technology, an appropriate set of input variables is known a priori. This is rarely the case in real applications. For example, in the process industries – a major target domain for neural network applications – plants are typically well instrumented and data is continuously collected from a large number of sensors.

We neural network practitioners sometimes claim that all available variables can be used; the learning algorithm will essentially ignore the irrelevant ones. This is not the whole truth. Superfluous variables place a burden on data collection that, in practice, can be infeasibly onerous. The greater the dimensionality of the input space, the greater the amount of data required for accurate modeling in general.

Correlations are a particular source of difficulty when extraneous inputs are employed. If undetected, correlated inputs can adversely affect the generalization properties of neural network models. Partial least squares (Wold 1966) addresses this problem by constructing the modeling relationship between projected principal component dimensions of the input and output vectors, rather than between the original (larger) input and output dimensions. An extension of PLS for nonlinear modeling has been developed based on neural networks (Qin and McAvoy 1992).

1.2.5. The Complexities of Neural Network Design.

The design space for neural networks is extraordinarily complex. In principle a neural network can have an arbitrary feedforward structure with each weight having its own learning rate parameter. Furthermore, the design criterion – what counts as a good neural network model – is application-dependent: depending on the problem, a different combination of criterion components such as learning speed, generalization accuracy, and network size may be important. As noted earlier, even the choice of model inputs is typically not obvious for real problems.

Yet the technology provides virtually no heuristic or analytic guidance to the application developer to allow her or him to deal with this complexity. The design approach that we perforce follow is a manual exploration limited to a small region of the potential design space. Thus all "reasonable" inputs are typically included, structures are limited to one or two hidden layers with full connectivity between adjacent layers, and one global learning rate is used. While good results can be obtained with effort, it is clear that the full potential of the technology is not being realized.

One approach to confronting the design complexity and taking advantage of the flexibility it offers is automated design. An optimization algorithm that has been used with some success in this context is a genetic algorithm. With a genetic algorithm, a search can be simultaneously conducted for an appropriate set of inputs, network structure, and learning algorithm parameters (Harp and Samad 1991 and 1994). Genetic algorithms are nongradient-based methods and make few assumptions about the problem. This is particularly helpful for neural network design since the optimization can be conducted over a combination of discrete and continuous dimensions and application-specific design criteria can be specified. In Harp and Samad (1994) an application to modeling the heat rate of the TVA Sequoyah nuclear power plant is described. The genetically optimized neural networks outperformed a sophisticated statistical model as well as hand-crafted neural networks.

1.3. Conclusions

This discussion has been limited to a selected few aspects of neural network application development. A more comprehensive treatment would include discussions of additional issues such as: adaptation in neural networks (the problem of incremental learning); the choice of optimization criterion for neural network learning; utilizing a priori knowledge (e.g., a rough first principles model) in neural network application development; selecting an appropriate neural network type (e.g., multilayer perceptrons or radial basis function networks); and the "black-box" criticism often leveled at neural networks.

In conclusion, one recurring theme in the discussion above bears re-articulation. There are numerous, and intimate, connections between neural networks and other technologies: many well-developed methods in statistics, system identification, and nonlinear optimization have direct relevance. Neural networks are not a technology unto themselves. It is by availing of synergies with conventional technologies that neural networks can revolutionize modeling applications.

1.4. References

Bryson, A.E. and Y.C. Ho, *Applied Optimal Control* (Hemisphere, 1975).

Fletcher, R. and C.M. Reeves, "Function minimization by conjugate gradients," *Computer Journal* **7** (1964) 149-154.

Geman, S., E. Bienenstock, and R. Doursat, "Neural networks and the bias/variance dilemma," *Neural Computation* **4** (1992) 1-58.

Harp, S.A. and T. Samad, "Genetic synthesis of neural network architecture," in *Handbook of Genetic Algorithms*, ed. L.D. Davis (Van Nostrand Reinhold, New York, 1991).

Harp, S.A. and T. Samad, "Genetic Optimization of Neural Network Architecture," *Tech. Report TR-104074* (Electric Power Research Institute, 3412 Hillview Avenue, Palo Alto, CA 94304, 1994).

Le Cun, Y., J.S. Denker, and S.A. Solla, "Optimal brain damage," in *Advances in Neural Information Processing Systems 2*, ed.s D.S. Touretzky (Morgan Kaufmann, 1990) pp. 598-605.

Leonard, J. and M.A. Kramer, "Improvement of the backpropagation algorithm for training neural networks," *Computers and Chemical Engineering* **14** (1990) 337-341.

Marquardt, D.W. "An algorithm for least-squares estimation for nonlinear parameters," *J. Soc. Ind. Appl. Math.* **11** (1963) 431-441.

Poggio, T. and F. Girosi, "Regularization algorithms for learning that are equivalent to multilayer networks," *Science* **247** (1990) 978-982.

Puskorius, G.V. and L.A. Feldkamp, "Neurocontrol of nonlinear dynamical systems with Kalman filter trained recurrent networks," *IEEE Transactions on Neural Networks* **5** (1994) 279-297.

Qin, S.J., and T.J. McAvoy, "Nonlinear PLC modeling using neural networks," *Computers and Chemical Engineering* **16** (1992) 379-391.

Sjöberg, J. and L. Ljung, "Overtraining, Regularization, and Searching for Minimum in Neural Networks," *Tech. Report LiTH-SY-I-1297* (Department of Electrical Engineering, Linköping University, S-581 83 Linköping, Sweden, 1992).

Su, H.T., T.J. McAvoy, and P.J. Werbos, "Long-term predictions of chemical processes using recurrent neural networks: a parallel training approach," *Industrial and Engineering Chemistry Research* **31** (1992) 1338-1352.

Werbos, P.J. "Backpropagation through time: what it is and how to do it," *Proceedings of the IEEE* **78** (1990) 1550-1560.

Wold, H., "Nonlinear estimation by iterative least squares procedures," in *Research Papers in Statistics*, ed. F. David (Wiley, New York, 1966)

2. PREDICTION HORIZON EFFECTS ON STOCHASTIC MODELING HINTS FOR NEURAL NETWORKS

RADU DROSSU AND ZORAN OBRADOVIĆ
School of Electrical Engineering and Computer Science, Washington State University
Pullman, Washington 99164-2752, USA
E-mail: rdrossu@eecs.wsu.edu, zoran@eecs.wsu.edu

ABSTRACT

The objective of this paper is to investigate the relationship between stochastic models and neural network (NN) approaches to time series modeling. Experiments on a complex real life prediction problem (entertainment video traffic) indicate that prior knowledge can be obtained through stochastic analysis both with respect to an appropriate NN architecture as well as to an appropriate sampling rate, in the case of a prediction horizon larger than one. An improvement of the obtained NN predictor is also proposed through a bias removal post-processing, resulting in much better performance than the best stochastic model.

2.1. Introduction

Time series prediction problems typically deal with either predicting a characteristic process parameter for the next time step (prediction horizon one), or with predicting a parameter several steps ahead (prediction horizon larger than one). Commonly, time series prediction problems are approached either from a stochastic perspective[2] or, more recently from a neural network (NN) perspective.[3,4] Each of these approaches has advantages and disadvantages: the stochastic methods are usually fast but limited in applicability since they usually employ linear models, whereas the NN methods are powerful enough but the choice of an appropriate architecture and parameters is a time consuming trial and error procedure. A combination of these two techniques either into a heterogeneous system or by applying a stochastic modeling for providing some prior knowledge for the NN learning hasn't been commonly dealt with.

The first objective of this work is to investigate whether a *hint* regarding an appropriate neural network architecture (to be more specific, number of external and context inputs) provided by stochastic modeling is valid. This hint would also indicate whether a feedforward or a recurrent NN is more appropriate for a given time series problem. An additional objective would be to investigate the relevance of a stochastic hint regarding an appropriate sampling rate for a given prediction horizon.

---

†This research was sponsored in part by the U.S. National Science Foundation (NSF) under research grant NSF-IRI-9308523.

2.2. ARMA Hints for Prediction Horizon One

In the case of a prediction horizon one, in which just the next value of the time series is predicted, the following stochastic hints were explored:

- whether an appropriate AR(p) model indicates the use of a feedforward NN with *p* external inputs;
- whether an appropriate MA(q) model indicates the use of a recurrent NN with *q* context inputs;
- whether an appropriate ARMA(p,q) model indicates the use of a recurrent NN with *p* external and *q* context inputs.

An additional context input is allowed in all cases to account for a possible first order differentiation used in the stochastic integrated model.

As a testbed, a complex real life prediction problem was used - compressed entertainment video traffic prediction. The results obtained indicated that the order of the stochastic model provided a good hint regarding the number of external and context inputs needed. They also indicated that, whereas the stochastic techniques performed better on preprocessed data (smoothed by applying a logarithmic transformation and stationarized by applying a first order differentiation), neural networks performed much better on raw data. The stochastic models provided an unbiased prediction; on the other hand, neural networks lead to biased predictors. A bias removal procedure was proposed that improved the neural network prediction significantly, outperforming the best stochastic models. A more detailed report on the prediction horizon one study will appear in Reference 1.

2.3. AR Hints for Larger Prediction Horizon

Since for a larger prediction horizon different sampling rates can be employed, the choice of an appropriate sampling rate based on the stochastic modeling is analyzed.

In addition, similar to the prediction horizon one, the following stochastic hint was explored:

- whether an appropriate AR(p) model indicates the use of a feedforward NN with *p* external inputs;

The same video traffic data was used for experimentation, but now with prediction horizon ten (the tenth step ahead process value is predicted). To predict the process $\hat{x}$ at time step t+10 using k process values up to time t, different sampling rates are considered:

- sampling rate 1, where the k previous process values are $x(t),x(t\text{-}1),x(t\text{-}2),\ldots,x(t\text{-}k+1)$;

- sampling rate 2, where the k previous process values are $x(t)$, $x(t\text{-}2)$, $x(t\text{-}4)$, ..., $x(t\text{-}2^*(k\text{-}1))$;
- sampling rate 5, where the k previous process values are $x(t)$, $x(t\text{-}5)$, $x(t\text{-}10)$, ..., $x(t\text{-}5^*(k\text{-}1))$;
- sampling rate 10, where the k previous process values are $x(t)$, $x(t\text{-}10)$, $x(t\text{-}20)$, ..., $x(t\text{-}10^*(k\text{-}1))$.

The performance of different AR models when sampling at rate 1 are shown in Table 2.1. Here the model was put into state space form and the Kalman filter was applied to obtain the predicted values. The error mean $\mu = \sum_1^n e_i / n$, the root mean squared error $RMSE = \sqrt{\sum_1^n e_i^2 / n}$ and the coefficient of determination $r^2 = 1 - MSE^2/VAR[x]$, where the e_i's stand for prediction errors and VAR[x] for the variance of the actual data and FPE stands for Akaike's Final Prediction Error. For a good predictor, the residuals should be normally distributed with μ close to 0, small MSE and r^2 close to 1 and the FPE should be maximal. The table suggests as most appropriate the AR(5) model, although there are just slight differences in performance between the AR(5), AR(6) and AR(7) models.

Table 2.1: Stochastic Models for Sampling Rate 1

Model	μ	**RMSE**	r^2	***FPE***
AR(2)	-1.639	534.648	0.667	0.004506
AR(3)	-1.641	534.648	0.667	0.004471
AR(4)	-1.639	534.649	0.667	0.004473
AR(5)	-1.635	534.640	0.667	0.004300
AR(6)	-1.643	534.657	0.667	0.004300
AR(7)	-1.658	534.644	0.667	0.004303
AR(8)	-1.670	534.662	0.667	0.004303
AR(9)	-1.658	534.658	0.667	0.004316

For the same sampling rate 1, the effect of different NN architectures on prediction accuracy is summarized in Tables 2.2 and 2.3. The results in Table 2.2 are obtained without postprocessing, whereas those in Table 2.3 are obtained by using the bias removal postprocessing mentioned earlier. The table indicates that the NN having 6 inputs yielded the best prediction this being consistent with the hint provided by the stochastic modeling (allowing an additional external input compared to the most appropriate AR(5) model to account for the first order differentiation).

The most appropriate AR models obtained for different sampling rates are presented in Table 2.4. The table indicates the sampling rate 1 as the most appropriate. For this particular sampling rate, the AR(5) model (using $x(t)$, $x(t\text{-}1)$, ..., $x(t\text{-}4)$ to predict $\hat{x}(t+10)$) yielded the best results.

Table 2.2: NN Architectures without Postprocessing

Architecture	μ	*RMSE*	r^2
3-3-1	-247.2198	666.3758	0.4920
4-4-1	-232.2317	653.1661	0.5135
5-5-1	-233.4985	652.2024	0.5158
6-6-1	-228.0229	649.8688	0.5204
7-7-1	-242.1205	653.9996	0.5152

Table 2.3: NN Architectures with Bias Removal Postprocessing

Architecture	μ	*RMSE*	r^2
3-3-1	-218.4767	656.2554	0.5074
4-4-1	-189.7234	639.2881	0.5339
5-5-1	-197.8836	640.3158	0.5333
6-6-1	-199.4722	640.4094	0.5342
7-7-1	-202.0774	640.2565	0.5354

Table 2.4: AR Models for Different Sampling Rates

Sampling	AR Order	μ	*RMSE*	r^2	*FPE*
1	5	-1.635	534.640	0.667	0.004300
2	4	4.042	544.573	0.442	0.006143
5	5	1.759	928.670	0.131	0.005720
10	4	31.118	855.588	0.361	0.013911

Table 2.5: NN Models for Different Sampling Rates

Sampling	Architecture	μ	*RMSE*	r^2
1	5-5-1	-197.8836	652.2024	0.5158
2	4-4-1	-172.9530	599.1706	0.4044
5	5-5-1	-26.0680	886.9009	0.2100
10	4-4-1	27.8088	870.7731	0.3326

The NN architectures corresponding to the best AR models for different sampling rates are given in Table 2.5 (except for the 4-4-1 architecture used with the sampling rate 10, all the prediction results are obtained after the application of the bias removal procedure). The results confirm the conclusion drawn from the stochastic analysis, according to which a sampling rate of 1 is the most appropriate.

2.4. Conclusions and Further Research

Experiments on the entertainment video time series with prediction horizon one indicated that a useful hint can be obtained through ARMA modeling regarding an appropriate NN architecture.

Preliminary results suggested that the hint is still valid for larger prediction horizons when using AR modeling. Useful information could also be gained from the stochastic analysis regarding an appropriate sampling rate.

The extension study from AR to ARMA modeling hints for larger prediction horizon is in progress. Further research is needed to explore the validity of these hints to other time series prediction problems.

2.5. References

1. R. Drossu and Z. Obradović, "Stochastic Modelling Hints for Neural Network Prediction," *Proc. of the World Congress on Neural Networks* (International Neural Network Society, Washington, DC, 1995).
2. G. Box and G. Jenkins, *Time Series Analysis: Forecasting and Control* (Prentice Hall, Englewood Cliffs, NJ, 1976).
3. P. Werbos, "Neural Networks, System Identification and Control in the Chemical Process Industries," in *Handbook of Intelligent Control, Neural, Fuzzy, and Adaptive Approaches* (Van Nostrand Reinhold, New York, 1992).
4. K.S. Narendra, "Adaptive Control of Dynamical Systems Using Neural Networks," in *Handbook of Intelligent Control, Neural, Fuzzy, and Adaptive Approaches* (Van Nostrand Reinhold, New York, 1992).

3. NEURAL NETWORK ANALYSIS FOR HAZARDOUS WASTE CHARACTERIZATION

MANAVENDRA MISRA, LORIEN Y. PRATT, C. FARRIS
Department of Mathematical and Computer Sciences, Center for Robotics and Intelligent Systems (CRIS), Colorado School of Mines
Golden, Colorado 80401-1887, USA
E-mail: mmisra@mines.colorado.edu, lpratt@mines.colorado.edu, cfarris@mines.colorado.edu

and

R.O. HANSEN
Department of Geophysics, Colorado School of Mines
Golden, Colorado 80401, USA
E-mail: rhansen@mines.colorado.edu

ABSTRACT

This paper is a summary of our work in developing a system for interpreting electromagnetic (EM) and magnetic sensor information from the dig face characterization experimental cell at Idaho National Engineering Laboratory (INEL) to determine the depth and nature of buried objects. This project contained three primary components: (1) development and evaluation of several geophysical interpolation schemes for correcting missing or noisy data, (2) development and evaluation of several wavelet compression schemes for removing redundancies from the data, and (3) construction of two neural networks that used the results of steps (1) and (2) to determine the depth and nature of buried objects. This work is a proof-of-concept study that demonstrates the feasibility of this approach. The resulting system was able to determine the nature of buried objects correctly 87% of the time and was able to locate a buried object to within an average error of 0.8 feet. These statistics were gathered based on a large test set and so can be considered reliable. Considering the limited nature of this study, these results strongly indicate the feasibility of this approach, and the importance of appropriate preprocessing of neural network input data.

3.1. Problem Background and Methodology

An estimated 2.1 million cubic meters of hazardous waste has been buried at a variety of U.S. Department of Energy (DOE) laboratories (Kostelnik 1993). This waste includes radioactive materials, toxic organics, and toxic heavy metals. Waste was sometimes dumped carelessly into open pits, which then accumulated water, causing the debris to shift. This material was also often stored in 208 liter (55

†This work was supported by Task Order 13, Master Task Subcontract Number C86-110877 from Idaho National Engineering Laboratory, Lockheed Idaho Technologies Co.

gallon) steel drums, which were crushed and shifted by construction equipment driven over the waste site.

An important step in remediating this waste is to characterize its position and shape before it is either dug up or treated in situ. Careful approaches to waste remediation require a precise characterization, so that disturbance to the waste can be minimized during remediation. This requirement may mean that only the uppermost portions of a waste site can be characterized adequately, so that an on-site *dig-characterize-dig* cycle is necessary. This scenario requires that data interpretation be fast, which implies that it be automated as much as possible, and that fast hardware be used in the automated part of the process.

There are a variety of geophysical methods that can be used to noninvasively detect buried waste. To maximize characterization accuracy, it seems appropriate to use multiple sensor types in a co-inversion process, where sensor data is converted to a map of the items being sensed.

This paper describes the performance of a system that uses electromagnetic (EM) and magnetic sensor data to determine the nature and depth of buried objects. Data is first corrected using a geophysical interpolation scheme, then compressed using a wavelet algorithm, then fed to two neural networks, which produce an estimate of the depth of a buried object, and a prediction about the type of object.

An important component of our work has been to evaluate principled preprocessing methods in order to clean up and reduce the amount of data that is fed to the neural networks. Cleaning up of the data amounts to using interpolation techniques to fill in missing data points, and to improve the signal to noise ratio of the data. A protocol to compare three of the interpolation algorithms most widely used in geophysics – minimum curvature, minimum curvature with smoothing, and kriging or least-squares collocation – was devised and executed. Once the decision had been made to use interpolation to reduce the data to a regularly-spaced grid, we decided to use wavelet transforms to compress the results of the interpolation. The transforms not only reduce the amount of data that will need to be input to the neural network, but also do a feature extraction so that the network can train quickly on just the important features in the data. It was decided to compare four wavelet families – Daubechies, Haar, Symmlet, and Coiflet – for this purpose. The purpose of the interpolation and wavelet transformations were to prepare the Dig Face data for depth and object type characterization of and location of subsurface objects.

The ability of neural networks to learn from sample input-output pairs makes them appropriate for the co-inversion task, where models for this process, especially as applied to real problems, are scarce. Examples of the input and output for this process are relatively cheap to obtain, however, by constructing forward models of various sensor types.

Neural networks are also attractive for this problem because they are readily implemented on parallel computers, which can drastically accelerate processing speed, and because they run quickly even on serial simulations of parallel hardware. The iterative dig face technique requires that the data for each level be processed quickly before moving on to the next level.

In the last few years, neural networks have begun to cross the boundary from research into deployment in profitable applications settings. For example applications, please see (Maren *et. al.* 1990). Neural networks have been applied by a number of researchers to the automated interpretation of geophysical data. By far the most thorough study on this subject is described by (Poulton *et. al.* 1992a, Poulton *et. al.* 1992b), who used back-propagation networks (Rumelhart*et. al.* 1987) to map electromagnetic (EM) data into offset, depth, and conductivity-area product, and compared back-propagation to several other neural network algorithms on this task, with favorable results.

As demonstrated in previous work, one reason that neural networks are an appropriate technology to explore for this problem is that they have been shown to do a good job at handling noisy data. In several empirical comparisons of neural networks to more traditional techniques, tasks which contained noisy data showed the largest improvement using a neural network approach (cf. (Fisher and McKusick 1989, Mooney *et. al.* 1989, Atlas *et. al.* 1990, Pratt and Norton 1990, Weiss and Kulikowski 1991, Shavlik *et. al.* 1991)).

3.2. Experimental Design and Results

The data supplied by INEL for this project consisted of the results of the six experiments conducted in the Dig Face Characterization Cell in 1993, described in (Josten 1993). As described in that report, the majority of the experiments consisted of measurements at a series of levels of vertical magnetic field intensity, vertical magnetic field gradient, horizontal and vertical dipole inphase and quadrature electromagnetic field measurements using a Geonics EM-38 instrument, and in some cases measurements from a volatile organic gas detector. Because the nature of the data acquired by the volatile organic gas detector is so different than that from the other sensors, no attempt was made to process the volatile organic gas data.

3.2.1. Interpolation

Interpolation was used to remedy the data of missing points, and to improve the signal to noise ratio in the data. A huge number of interpolation algorithms for multi-dimensional data exist. It was decided to concentrate on a careful comparison of a few algorithms on the selected data. The three algorithms chosen are:

1. Minimum Curvature Interpolation: It is possible to implement minimum-curvature interpolation in a number of ways. The software used in this project, MINCL, is a modification of the program published by (Webring 1981), which is based on the technique suggested by (Briggs 1974).
2. Minimum Curvature Interpolation with Smoothing: This technique is a modification of the minimum curvature method which takes into account the possible presence of noise in the data. The software used for this project was GCV (Bates *et. al.* 1990).
3. Kriging or Least Squares Collocation: Kriging (Matheron 1963) and least-squares collocation (Moritz 1978) are essentially identical interpolation methods (Hardy 1984). The software used for this technique was KGRID (Hansen 1993).

These techniques are probably by far the most commonly used in exploration geophysics; as the exploration geophysics community makes extensive use of interpolation this is probably a reasonable selection criterion.

These data were then systematically degraded, and each of the interpolation programs were run on the degraded data. To simulate missing data, random numbers were drawn from a uniform bi-dimensional distribution with bounds equal to the limits of the data distribution to determine which points to remove. Drawing continued until a pre-set fraction of the data points had been deleted. The levels of missing data ranged from 5 to 60%. To simulate noise, random numbers drawn from a Gaussian distribution whose variance was a fixed fraction of the data variance for that variable were added to each data value. The ratios of the variances ranged from 5 to 60%. The three interpolation algorithms were then used to reconstruct from the degraded data, and the reconstruction was compared with the baseline clean data using root-mean-square error. These experiments were run both for the missing data case, as well as the noise degradation case.

Results: The two minimum curvature algorithms are consistently better than the kriging algorithm in reconstructing missing data, but there is otherwise little to choose between them. For noise-contaminated data, GCV outperformed the other two programs.

To test for the possibility that the comparison between the interpolation algorithms was being influenced by outliers, a second set of comparisons was made using the supremum norm rather than the root mean square norm (i.e., finding the maximum absolute values of the deviations between the interpolated results and the reference data, rather than the root mean square deviations). The results were substantially the same as for the RMS differences.

It should be noted that the relative running times of the three algorithms varied dramatically: an average interpolation run required 30 seconds on an IBM RS/6000 for MINCL, 15 minutes for GCV and 18 minutes for KGRID. This reflects much optimization of the MINCL program for production use (Webring 1981).

Despite the run-time performance penalty, we would recommend the GCV program on the basis of its excellent noise rejection capability. An additional feature of this program, is that it supports three-dimensional interpolation.

3.2.2. Wavelet Transforms

There is a wide acceptance that preprocessing neural network input data is a good idea, especially when it is of high dimension (Hertz *et. al.* 1991, Minsky and Papert 1969). Networks for dig face data interpretation will need to process extremely large amounts of input information. In such cases, it is desirable to reduce the amount of data to a minimal set that retains the salient features of the original data. This reduced data set can then form the input to a neural network, or to other algorithms for characterizing object depth and characteristics. For a neural network, the removal of redundancies in the data afforded by data compression speeds up training time and improves the trained network's performance.

Wavelet transforms have recently emerged as a sound technique for data compression (Strang 1994). These transforms represent the signal of interest in the form of coefficients corresponding to a basis consisting of a family of wavelet functions. The proper choice of the wavelet family leads to a representation where a majority of the coefficients are below some threshold. Compression of the signal can therefore be achieved by retaining only those coefficients that are larger than the threshold and discarding the rest. These transforms have been used for compression of fingerprint images, compression of signals to be transmitted, and various kinds of image analysis.

A decision was made to empirically test the performance of four families of discrete wavelet transforms (Haar, Daubechies, Symmlet, and Coiflet) in compressing the dig face data. In addition to the wavelet transforms, as a baseline test each data set was also compressed using decimation on a 2-D FFT of the data set. We measured the performance of each class of wavelets by varying the amount of compression for each class, and reporting the RMS error from the reconstructions of the data image, in a similar manner to the technique used for comparing the performance of various interpolation methods.

Results: All the wavelet transforms outperformed the FFT as a compression method, especially at higher compression levels. At low levels of compression (i.e. 25% of the data retained), the wavelet transforms tended to perform equally well. However, at high levels of compression, only those transforms with many coefficients were able to create good reconstructions. Twenty coefficients simply store more information in the transform itself than twelve or sixteen coefficients. For this reason, Daubechies-20 was selected as the wavelet transform to be used in the next stage of the project.

3.2.3. Neural Networks

The goal of this project was to construct a system that would locate and characterize the nature of buried objects, using sensor data representing six different modalities: vertical magnetic field intensity, vertical magnetic field gradient, EM horizontal in-phase, EM vertical in-phase, EM horizontal quadrature, and EM vertical quadrature. To achieve this goal, two neural networks were constructed: the characterization *network* and the *depth network*. The characterization network predicts the nature of material in the center four grid positions of the input, while the depth network produces a single real-valued number representing the network's estimate of the depth of a buried object.

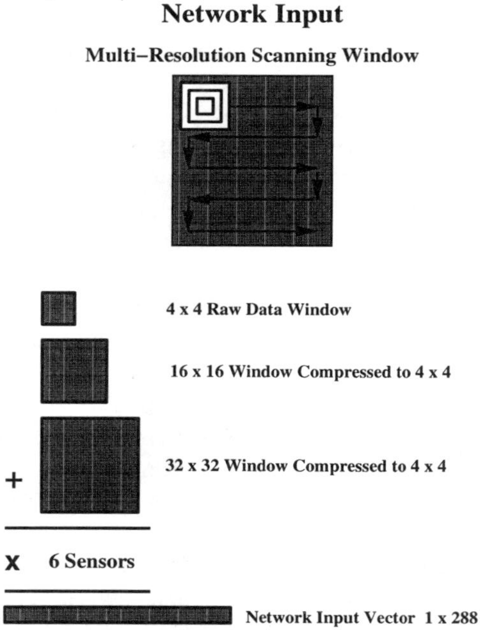

Figure 3.1. A representation of the multi-resolution input to the neural networks.

Input to both networks are from a multi-resolution scan of the input (preprocessed) data. At each position, the networks receive a 4×4 window of raw data, a 16×16 window is wavelet compressed to 4×4, and a 32×32 window is also wavelet compressed to 4×4 (Figure 3.1). Thus, the networks receive high resolution data from the immediate vicinity of a point, and successively lower resolution information about points further away. The networks were trained on extremely large training sets, and a separate validation set is used to determine when to stop training without overfitting. Finally, the networks are tested on a completely separate testing set.

Results: The neural network experiments are still ongoing. However, the preliminary results are encouraging. The characterization net performed at 87% accuracy, and the depth net identifies the depth of a buried object within an average error of 0.8 feet. There are a number of efforts underway that will doubtless improve the performance of both networks.

3.3. Conclusions

We have evaluated three interpolations schemes and recommend the use of GCV for the dig face data. Likewise, our experiments lead us to recommend Daubechies-20 as the wavelet transform best suited to compress this data. Our work shows that principled data preprocessing is critical in order to speedup training, and increase accuracy of neural network performance. Finally, we have shown the feasibility of applying neural networks to the site characterization problem, especially when data from multiple sensors has to be fused to obtain an accurate prediction.

3.4. Acknowledgments

CSM undergraduate student Jeremy Bargen and graduate student Altaf Siddiqui helped with neural network training in the spring of 1995. Their assistance both in running neural networks and also in providing input to this document was invaluable.

3.5. References

L.E. Atlas, J. Connor, D. Park, A. Lippman, R. Cole, M. El-Sharkawi, R.J. Marks, Y. Muthusamy and M. Rudnick, "A Performance Comparison of Trained Multi-Layer Perceptrons and Trained Classification Trees," in *IEEE International Conference on Systems, Man, and Cybernetics* (IEEE, Piscataway, NJ, 1990).

D.M. Bates, F. Reames and G. Wahba, "Getting better contour plots with S and GCVPACK," *Technical Report 865* (University of Wisconsin, 1990).

I.C. Briggs, "Machine contouring using minimum curvature," *Geophysics* **39** (1974) 39-48.

Douglas H. Fisher and Kathleen B. McKusick, "An Empirical Comparison of ID3 and Back-propagation," in Proceedings of the Eleventh International Joint

Conference on Artificial Intelligence (Morgan Kaufmann, Detroit, MI 1989), pp. 788-793.

R.O. Hansen, "Interpretative gridding by anisotropic kriging," *Geophysics* **58** (1993) 1491-1497.

R.L. Hardy, "Kriging, collocation and biharmonic models for applications in the earth sciences (what's the difference)," *Technical Papers of the American Congress of Surveying and Mapping* **44** (1984) 363-372.

John A. Hertz and Richard G. Palmer and Anders S. Krogh, *Introduction to the theory of neural computation* (Addison-Wesley, Redwood City, CA, 1991), pg. 144

N.E. Josten, "A New Application for Geophysics: Monitoring at the Dig-face During Waste Site Excavation," in *Symposium on the Application of Geophysics to Engineering and Environmental Problems*, Vol. 1, ed.s Ronald S. Bell and C. Melvin Lepper (Environmental and Engineering Geophysical Society, San Diego, CA, 1993), pp. 301-317.

K.M. Kostelnik, "Buried Waste Integrated Demonstration Strategy Plan," *Technical Report EGG-WTD-10610* (Idaho National Engineering Laboratory, Idaho Falls, ID, 1993).

Allianna J. Maren, Craig T. Harston and Robert M. Pap, *Handbook of neural computing applications* (Academic Press, San Diego, CA, 1990).

G. Matheron, "Principles of geostatistics," *Economic Geology* **58** (1963) 1246-1266.

Marvin L. Minsky and Seymour A. Papert, *Perceptrons* (The MIT Press, Cambridge, MA, 1969).

Raymond J. Mooney, J.W. Shavlik, G.G. Towell and A. Gove, "An Experimental Comparison of Symbolic and Connectionist Learning Algorithms," in *Proceedings of the Eleventh International Joint Conference on Artificial Intelligence* (Morgan Kaufmann, San Mateo, CA, 1989).

H. Moritz, "Least-squares collocation," Reviews of Geophysics and Space Physics **16** (1978) 27-36.

M.M. Poulton, B.K. Sternberg and C.E. Glass, "Neural network pattern recognition of subsurface EM images," *Journal of Applied Geophysics* **29** (1992) 21-36.

Mary M. Poulton, Ben K. Sternberg and Charles E. Glass, "Location of subsurface targets in geophysical data using neural networks," *Geophysics* **57** (1992) 1534-1544.

Lorien Y. Pratt and Steve W. Norton, "Neural Networks and Decision Tree Induction: Exploring the relationship between two research areas," in *Workshop Summary, Neural Information Processing Systems* (1990).

D.E. Rumelhart, G.E. Hinton and R.J. Williams, "Learning Internal Representations by Error Propagation," in *Parallel Distributed Processing: Explorations in the*

Microstructure of Cognition, Vol. 1, ed.s David E. Rumelhart and James L. McClelland (MIT Press: Bradford Books, 1987), pp. 318-362.

J.W. Shavlik, R.J. Mooney and G.G. Towell, "Symbolic and Neural Net Learning Algorithms: An Experimental Comparison," *Machine Learning* **6(2)** (1991) 111-143.

Gilbert Strang, "Wavelets," *American Scientist* **82** (1994) 250-255.

M. Webring, "Minc, a gridding program based on minimum curvature," *Open File Report 81-1224* (U.S. Geological Survey, 1981).

Sholom M. Weiss and Casimir A. Kulikowski, *Computer Systems that Learn* (Morgan Kaufmann, San Mateo, CA, 1991).

4. NEURAL NETWORKS FOR NUCLEAR SPECTROSCOPY

PAUL E. KELLER, LARS J. KANGAS, SHERIF HASHEM
Pacific Northwest National Laboratory†, P.O. Box 999, MS K1-87
Richland, Washington 99352, USA
E-mail: pe_keller@pnl.gov, lj_kangas@pnl.gov

RICHARD T. KOUZES
Department of Physics, West Virginia University, P.O. Box 6216, 302 Stewart Hall
Morgantown, West Virginia 26505, USA
E-mail: rkouzes@wvnvm.wvnet.edu

and

GARY L. TROYER,
Westinghouse Hanford Company††, P.O. Box 1970, MS T6-50
Richland, Washington 99352, USA
E-mail: gary_l_troyer@rl.gov

ABSTRACT

In this paper two applications of artificial neural networks (ANNs) in nuclear spectroscopy analysis are discussed. In the first application, an ANN assigns quality coefficients to alpha particle energy spectra. These spectra are used to detect plutonium contamination in the work environment. The quality coefficients represent the levels of spectral degradation caused by miscalibration and foreign matter affecting the instruments. A set of spectra was labeled with quality coefficients by an expert and used to train the ANN expert system. Our investigation shows that the expert knowledge of spectral quality can be transferred to an ANN system.

The second application combines a portable gamma-ray spectrometer with an ANN. In this system the ANN is used to automatically identify radioactive isotopes in real-time from their gamma-ray spectra. Two neural network paradigms are examined: the linear perceptron and the optimal linear associative memory (OLAM). A comparison of the two paradigms shows that OLAM is superior to linear perceptron for this application. Both networks have a linear response and are useful in determining the composition of an unknown sample when the spectrum of the unknown is a linear superposition of known spectra. One feature of this technique is that it uses the whole spectrum in the identifica-

---

†This work was supported by the Laboratory Directed Research and Development Program and by the Environmental Molecular Sciences Laboratory construction project at Pacific Northwest National Laboratory (PNNL). PNNL is a multiprogram national laboratory operated by Battelle Memorial Institute for the U.S. Department of Energy under Contract DE-AC06-76RLO 1830.
††Westinghouse Hanford Company is the Hanford Operations Contractor for the U.S. Department of Energy under Contract DE-AC06-87RL10930.

tion process instead of only the individual photo-peaks. For this reason, it is potentially more useful for processing data from lower resolution gamma-ray spectrometers. This approach has been successfully tested with data generated by Monte Carlo simulations and with field data from both sodium iodide and germanium detectors.

With the ANN approach, the intense computation takes place during the training process. Once the network is trained, normal operation consists of propagating the data through the network, which results in rapid identification of samples. This approach is useful in situations that require fast response but where precise quantification is less important.
Keywords: artificial neural networks, nuclear spectroscopy, isotope identification, gamma-ray, alpha particle.

4.1. Introduction

Enormous amounts of hazardous waste were generated by more than 40 years of plutonium production at the U.S. Department of Energy's Hanford site. There are an estimated 1700 waste sites distributed around the 1450 square kilometers of southeastern Washington state that comprise this site.[1] This waste includes nuclear waste (e.g., fission products), toxic chemical waste (e.g., carbon tetrachloride, ferrocyanide, nitrates, etc.), and mixed waste (combined radioactive and chemical waste). The Pacific Northwest National Laboratory is exploring the technologies required to perform environmental restoration and waste management in a cost-effective manner. This includes the development of compact, portable, and inexpensive systems capable of real-time identification of contaminants. The objective of our research is to demonstrate the potential information processing capabilities of the neural network paradigm in real-time, automated identification of contaminants.

ANNs are used in a wide variety of data processing applications where real-time data analysis and information extraction are required. One advantage of this approach is that most of the intense computation takes place during the training process. Once the ANN is trained for a particular task, operation is relatively fast and spectra can be rapidly processed. Another feature of this approach is that human intervention is not required during system operation which promotes automation. An ANN coupled to a sensing system, such as a spectrometer, can be used as a portable, automated system for identifying contaminants. In this paper, ANNs are applied to two applications: one for identifying quality of alpha spectra and another for identifying isotopes from their gamma-ray spectra.

4.2. Alpha Spectral Quality Assignment

Air quality monitoring for man-made alpha emitting radioisotopes in nuclear processing and storage facilities is performed by measurement of collected particulates on air filters. The filters collect fine dust particles including naturally occurring alpha emitters. The filters are observed in real time by alpha spectrometers which create energy spectra. As dust or overmass builds on the filter, the spectral resolution and the ability to differentiate isotopes of interest is compromised.

A desirable goal is to take corrective action before a spectrum degrades past usefulness. With significant experience, an operator can determine the usefulness of an alpha spectrum by visual inspection. In the case of too much overmass, a simple non-scheduled filter change cycle is performed. In other cases, poor spectral quality may indicate that detector or electronic maintenance is required. Regardless, intervention in the measurement system is required. However, the dynamics of facility operations preclude constant watch of spectral accumulations in real time. Thus, automated early warning based on spectral quality can assure that an isotope of concern is being reliably monitored.

The possibility of using an automated ANN approach to provide real-time inference was proposed as an alternative to more common methods.[2] Many investigators have attempted to maintain spectral quality through system design or special algorithms.[3] All are limited by the reality of dynamic operations and the potential for unexpected and rapid spectral degradation. Some empirical numerical tests have been performed which are complex *a posteriori* exercises. None of the methods have proved attractive for real-time application.

4.3. Approach

The first investigation was performed on 139 alpha particle spectra received from Westinghouse Hanford Company. The spectra were generated to identify the presence of airborne plutonium in work environments. Minute levels of plutonium are easily lost in the background noise from degraded alpha emitting progeny of radon gas. In order to identify plutonium, these spectra must be of high quality.

ANNs were applied to the problem of assessing the degradation in the quality of the alpha spectra, a task that is presently performed by human experts. Experts use graphical representations of spectra during assessments. The ANN technology was chosen because it has the same capability as experts in analyzing spectral channels in parallel. ANNs have demonstrated their benefits in other applications of spectral analysis.[4-7]

The spectra used in this investigation showed various levels of quality degradation due to variables such as calibration and salt build-up on the filter used in counting the alpha particles. Each spectrum was labeled with a quality coefficient from 0 to 10 by an expert. The spectra labeled from 0 to 3 are acceptable for determining plutonium levels. The labels in the midrange (4-6) are marginally acceptable. High labels, above 6, indicate poor quality spectra and that the filter needs replacement and/or that the instrument needs calibration. Figure 4.1 illustrates 2 of the spectra. The task for the ANN was to learn to label spectra with quality coefficients using the knowledge of a human expert.

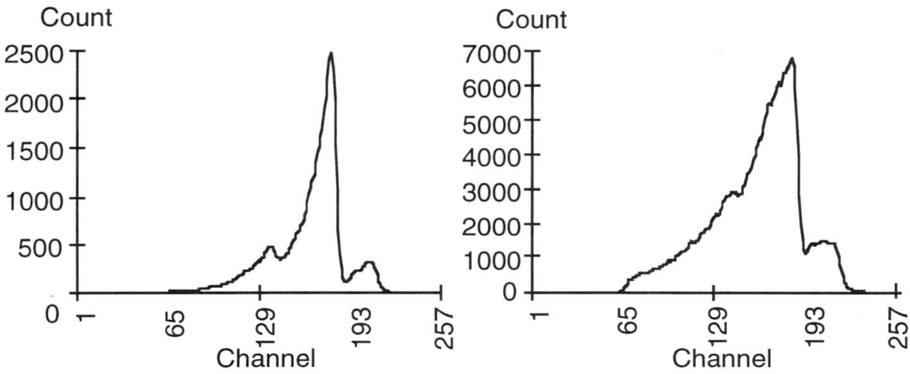

(a) (b)

Figure 4.1. Alpha spectra. (a) Optimal spectra with an expert assessed quality coefficient of 1. (b) Degraded spectra with an expert assessed quality coefficient of 5. Observe that the differences in the scale of the vertical axis are insignificant. The vertical axis represent energy count and is not analyzed as absolute values.

The original alpha spectra were sampled at 512 channels and reduced to 256 channels during the data collection. During our initial data analysis, it was observed that all the spectral information was found between channels 40 and 239. These 200 channels were further processed to reduce the amount of data being fed into the ANN as shown in Figure 4.2. The 200 channels were reduced into 20 equal sized channels, with each new channel computed as the average of 10 consecutive channels. This reduction in the spectral resolution was deemed appropriate for the relatively few spectra used in this investigation. The channel counts in each spectrum were normalized to the maximum channel count of the spectrum before presentation to the ANN.

The ANN used to qualify the alpha spectra is illustrated in Figure 4.3. The network consisted of 20 inputs for the averaged spectral values, one hidden layer with 15 nodes, and one output node for the spectral quality value. The ANNs were trained using the standard backpropagation algorithm with batch mode weight updates.[8] The learning rate and momentum were kept constant at 0.01 and 0.9, respectively. The training of the ANNs was stopped at 3000 epochs. This ANN configuration and these training variables had been previously determined to yield near optimal performance.

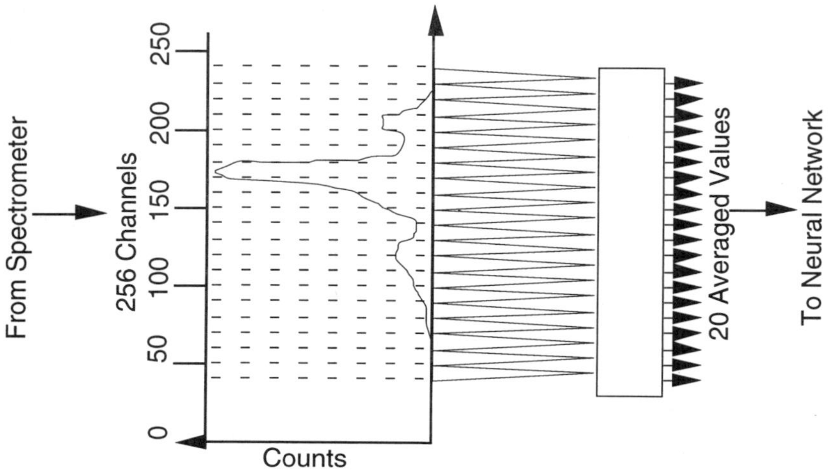

Figure 4.2. Preprocessing of the 256 spectral channels reduces the number of values to 20.

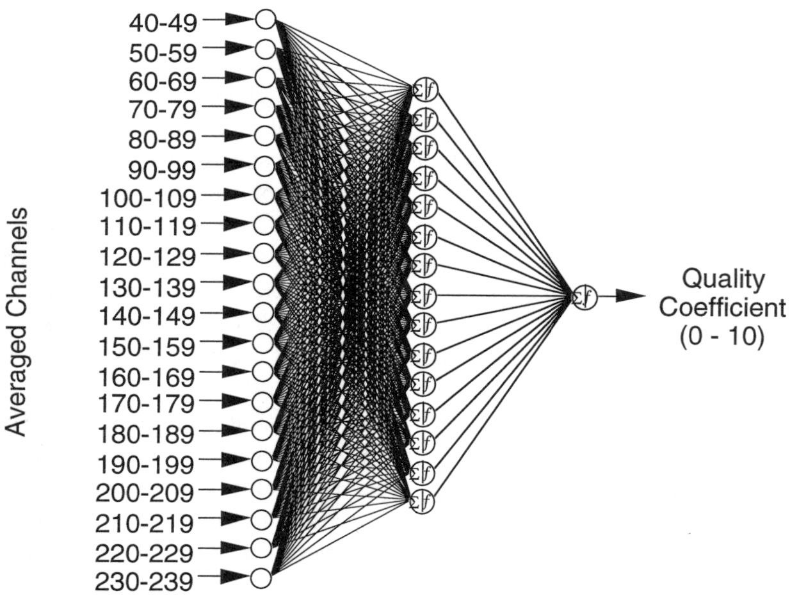

Figure 4.3. ANN with 20 spectral values as inputs and one output which is the assessed quality coefficient for the spectrum being analyzed. The figure shows that only the values from channels 40 to 239 of the 256 channel spectra are input to the ANN.

4.4. Alpha Spectra Quality Assignment Results and Discussion

The performance of an ANN is evaluated with testing data. An unbiased evaluation requires that these testing data are separate from the data used in training. In order to test all spectra available for this investigation, we partitioned the spectra into four equal sized sets and used the K-fold testing approach. Each set was tested using a separate ANN that was trained with the other three sets. By using four ANNs and rotating the set used for testing, all spectra in the four testing sets were labeled. The K-fold testing approach resulted in an RMS error of 1.252 (MSE = 1.567) measured over all data (which has a range of 0 to 10).

Our investigation shows that the expert knowledge of spectral quality can be transferred to an ANN system. The histogram in Figure 4.4 shows that only a small fraction of the spectra on hand have significant errors. Most spectra were qualified by the ANN system to be within ±2 coefficient values from those assigned by the expert. The deviation is within ±1 for 83.5% of the spectra and within ±2 for 97.1%.

It is further noted that where extreme deviations existed, information in the spectra was not included in the expert's coefficient assignment. In particular, the worst mismatch had good spectral quality but included an additional isotope signal not in the majority of training spectra. Thus, it is expected that inclusion of a second condition for indicating the presence of the interfering isotope would improve the variance while providing an indicator of isotopic presence as an important side benefit.

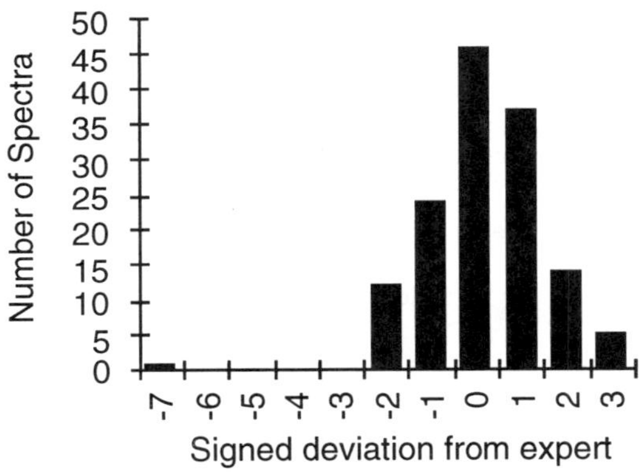

Figure 4.4. Distribution of deviation from expert. The figure shows the signed deviation (ANN - Expert) of the ANN assessed quality coefficients from the expert's coefficients.

4.5. Gamma-Ray Isotope Identification

The traditional approach to isotope identification from gamma-ray spectra can be categorized as finding peaks and fitting curves. This approach involves an iterative process of spectrum decomposition and regeneration until a mathematically synthesized spectrum closely matching the true spectrum can be generated. This is both time consuming and often requires manual intervention. The ANN approach employs pattern recognition on the entire spectrum. This recognition is performed by a single vector-matrix multiplication that results in rapid, real-time identification of analytes and can be used in automated systems.

For a sample composed of a combination of isotopes, the spectrum of the sample, $\underline{S}$, is approximately a linear superposition of the spectra of each individual isotope, $\underline{s}_i$. This is illustrated by Eq. (4.1) where α_i is the relative concentration of each isotope in the sample:

$$\underline{S} = \sum_i \alpha_i \underline{s}_i . \tag{4.1}$$

Therefore, the classification system should have a linear response with respect to the input. This deviates from the majority of ANN applications, such as the previous one, which implement a nonlinear response. However, even with a linear response, the ANN approach has advantages in speed, simplicity, and automation over traditional approaches.

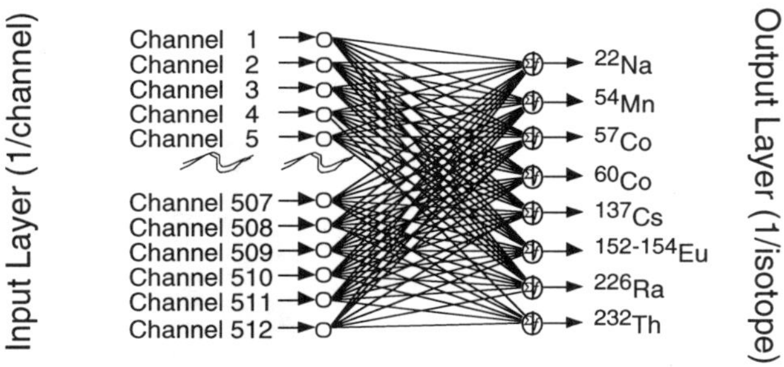

Figure 4.5. An ANN used to identify radioactive isotopes.

An ANN designed to have a linear response employs linear activation functions. A feedforward ANN that implements linear activation functions can be reduced to a network with a single input layer and single output layer. Therefore, the ANN used in this application has a single input and single output layer as illustrated in Figure 4.5. Two ANN paradigms were studied for implementing the linear response: the linear perceptron and the optimal linear associative memory. Both approaches to gamma-ray spectral analysis have been applied separately.[9-12] In this paper, these two ANN techniques are compared.

4.5.1. Linear Perceptron

Linear perceptron is one of the oldest ANN paradigms. It originally sparked interest in the pattern recognition community in the late 1950s and early 1960s.[13] However, it was unable to solve pattern recognition problems that were not linearly separable. The original perceptron implemented a hard-limited threshold as the activation function. For the gamma-ray spectral analysis application, a modified linear activation function (linear for positive input and zero for negative input) known as a perceptron function is used. The delta rule is used to train the perceptron in an iterative process, which is detailed in Table 4.1. With linear activation functions, this training algorithm is mathematically identical to the backpropagation algorithm[8] since the derivative terms in backpropagation would be unity in this case.

Table 4.1: Perceptron Learning Rule

Step 1.	Initialize weights with random values.
Step 2.	Pick a labeled pattern (spectrum, $\underline{x}^p$, and known composition, $\underline{t}^p$) from the training set and present the spectrum to the network.
Step 3.	Propagate data forward and generate the output classification. $\underline{y}^p = \underline{\underline{W}}\, \underline{x}^p$
Step 4.	Calculate mean-square error between target classification and actual classification.
Step 5.	Adapt the synaptic weights by using a delta rule to reduce output error. $\Delta\underline{\underline{W}} = \eta(\underline{t}^p - \underline{y}^p)\underline{x}^p$ (η = learning rate)
Step 6.	If there are more spectra in the training set, loop back to step 2.
Step 7.	If the output error is high or the maximum number of iterations have not been met, then loop back to step 2.

4.5.2. Optimal Linear Associative Memory (OLAM)

The optimal linear associative memory (OLAM) approach is based on a simple matrix associative memory model.[14,15] It was developed in the early 1970s as a content addressable memory and is useful in situations where the input consists of a linear combination of known patterns (e.g., gamma-ray spectra). It is an improvement over the original matrix memory approach in that it projects an input pattern onto a set of orthogonal vectors where each orthogonal vector represents a unique pattern (exemplar). With linear activation functions, the training is a straight forward matrix orthogonalization process where each pattern from the training set is made to project onto a separate, unique orthogonal axis in the output space. This process is described in Table 4.2.

Table 4.2: OLAM Weight Specification

Step 1.	Form matrices of spectra and isotopic concentrations. Arrange spectra, $\underline{x}^p$, as columns in an n×p dimensional matrix $\underline{\underline{X}}$ and target concentrations, $\underline{t}^p$, as columns in an m×p dimensional matrix $\underline{\underline{T}}$.
Step 2.	Generate inverse of the spectral matrix $\underline{\underline{X}}$. Since $\underline{\underline{X}}$ is generally not a square matrix, a pseudo-inverse technique is used to generate $\underline{\underline{X}}^\dagger$. († indicates pseudo-inverse)
Step 3.	Form the synaptic weight matrix. $\underline{\underline{W}} = \underline{\underline{TX}}^\dagger$

4.6. Isotope Identification System Layout

Figure 4.6 illustrates a prototype system that combines a portable gamma-ray spectrometer with an ANN. Figure 4.5 illustrates the ANN that is connected to the gamma-ray spectrometer. In this prototype, a sodium iodide (NaI) detector is used, and 512 channels of data are produced by the spectrometer. All channels are fed into the ANN so that there is one input for every channel. There is a single processing layer (output layer) in the ANN where the number of output neurons is equal to the number of isotopes being identified (8 in this case). One feature of this approach to gamma-ray spectral analysis is that the whole spectrum is used in the identification process instead of individual peaks in the spectrum. For this reason, it is potentially more useful for processing data from lower resolution gamma-ray spectrometers like those employing NaI detectors.

Each isotope presented to the spectrometer produces a spectrum that is characteristic of that isotope. By presenting many different isotopes to the system, a database of spectra is constructed. From this database, training sets and test sets are generated. These sets are collections of labeled patterns (spectra of isotopes with known concentrations) representative of the desired identification mapping. The training sets are used to configure the ANN. The goal of this training is to learn an association between the spectra and the labels representing the spectra. ANNs were developed with both the linear perceptron learning rule and with the OLAM weight specification. The training process for the OLAM is a non-iterative process, while the linear perceptron training process requires thousands of iterations. For this reason, it took only 200 milliseconds on a SPARCstation 10 to generate the OLAM ANN, while it took a couple of hours to generate the linear perceptron ANN. Training times on an Intel i486 based personal computer are only a few times greater than this.

4.7. Gamma Spectra Results

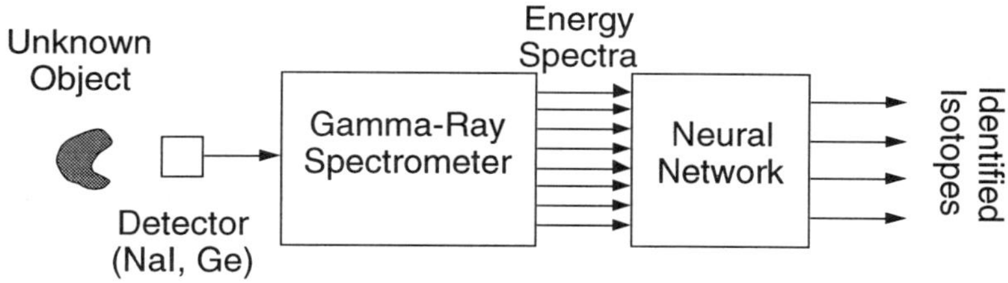

Figure 4.6. Prototype system combining gamma-ray spectrometer with an ANN.

The prototype system illustrated in Figure 4.6 was tested with both Monte Carlo simulated spectra and field data collected from a gamma spectrometer equipped with a sodium iodide detector. Figure 4.5 illustrates the ANN configured to identify 8 radioactive isotopes (^{22}Na, ^{54}Mn, ^{57}Co, ^{60}Co, ^{137}Cs, $^{152\text{-}154}$Eu, ^{226}Ra, and ^{232}Th) from their gamma-ray spectra. Field operation consists of presenting an unknown sample to the system, generating a gamma-ray spectrum, passing the spectrum through the ANN, and generating a classification of the unknown sample. The values on the output neurons are proportional to the quantities of each radioactive isotope found in the sample. Figure 4.7 illustrates the classification of a sample composed of equal amounts of ^{60}Co and ^{137}Cs (sample 4). In this case, the OLAM correctly identified the composition of the samples while the linear perceptron incorrectly identified a significant amount of ^{57}Co. Figure 4.8 illustrates the classification of a sample composed of equal amounts of ^{22}Na, ^{57}Co, ^{60}Co, ^{137}Cs, and $^{152\text{-}154}$Eu (sample 5). In this case the OLAM correctly identifies all the isotopes present in the sample though the ratios between identified isotopes are not uniform. The linear perceptron had a hard time identifying ^{60}Co and often identified ^{57}Co when it was not present. Figure 4.9 illustrates the classification of a sample composed of equal amounts of ^{22}Na, ^{60}Co, ^{137}Cs, and $^{152\text{-}154}$Eu (sample 7). In this case, the OLAM incorrectly identified a small amount of ^{54}Mn while the linear perceptron did not identify the presence of ^{60}Co and misidentified a small amount of ^{54}Mn. The linear perceptron had a hard time identifying ^{60}Co and often identified ^{57}Co when it was not present. In several additional cases, the OLAM indicated a small amount of ^{54}Mn when it was not present. However, the errors with the OLAM were always smaller than the linear perceptron. Similar results were found with other samples which can be found in Table 4.3. Additional studies that were performed with a Germanium detector yielded similar results.

Table 4.4 lists results from Monte Carlo simulated spectra. The linear perceptron and OLAM were tested on spectra of mixtures and on modified spectra. Spectra of mixtures were generated by combining the simulated spectra of the different isotopes. Modified spectra were produced by reducing the peak height of some spectra and by removing everything but the peak of other spectra. Since both the spectrum of the mixtures and the OLAM were generated from ideal spectra, the OLAM perfectly identified all the isotopes in the different mixtures. The linear perceptron did not fair well. For the modified spectra, the linear perceptron performed slightly better than the OLAM. These results indicate that the linear perceptron uses the peak information more than the OLAM does.

The time to identify an isotope from a 512 channel spectrum with 8 possible isotopes is 20 milliseconds on a 33 MHz Intel *i*486DX based personal computer. Therefore, the classification process is limited not by the ANN but by the time it takes to acquire and generate a spectrum. In applications that can acquire and deliver data much faster, the ANN can be implemented in specialized hardware. In such a case, three orders of magnitude increase in classification speed can be achieved.

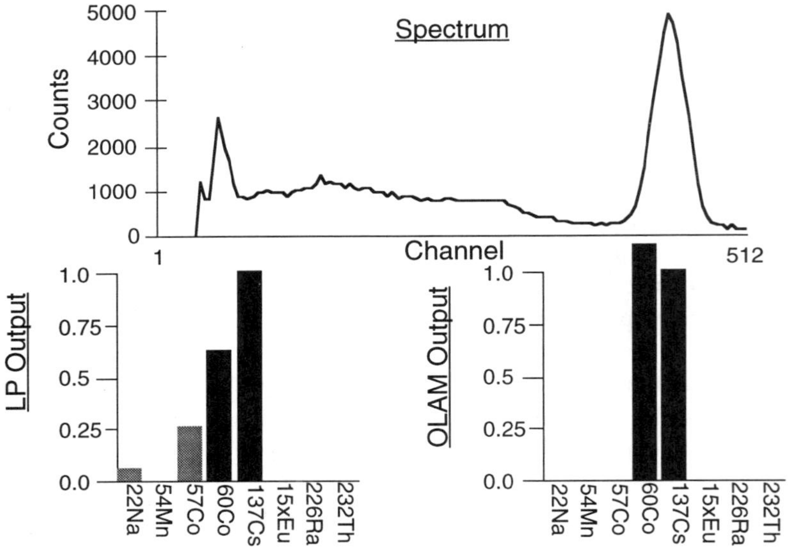

Figure 4.7. Spectrum of a mixture of ^{60}Co and ^{137}Cs (sample 4) with the associated classifications by the linear perceptron (LP) and OLAM ANNs. ANN outputs in gray indicate incorrect identification of an isotope.

4.8. Conclusions

The results of our research have demonstrated the benefits of the neural network paradigm in analyzing spectral data. Some of its advantages over conventional analytical techniques include simplicity, real-time analysis, and the absence of human intervention. All of these are important in building compact and portable systems for automated contaminant identification.

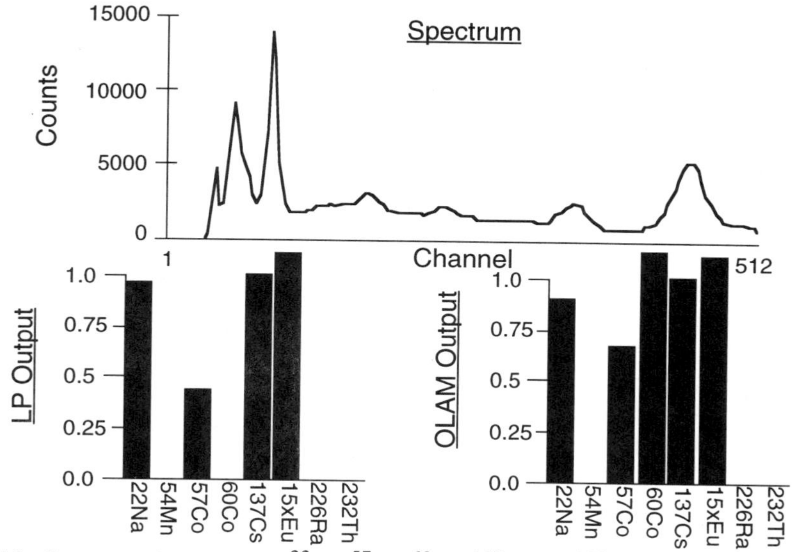

Figure 4.8. Spectrum of a mixture of ^{22}Na, ^{57}Co, ^{60}Co, ^{137}Cs and $^{152\text{-}154}Eu$ (sample 5) with the associated classifications by the linear perceptron (LP) and OLAM ANNs.

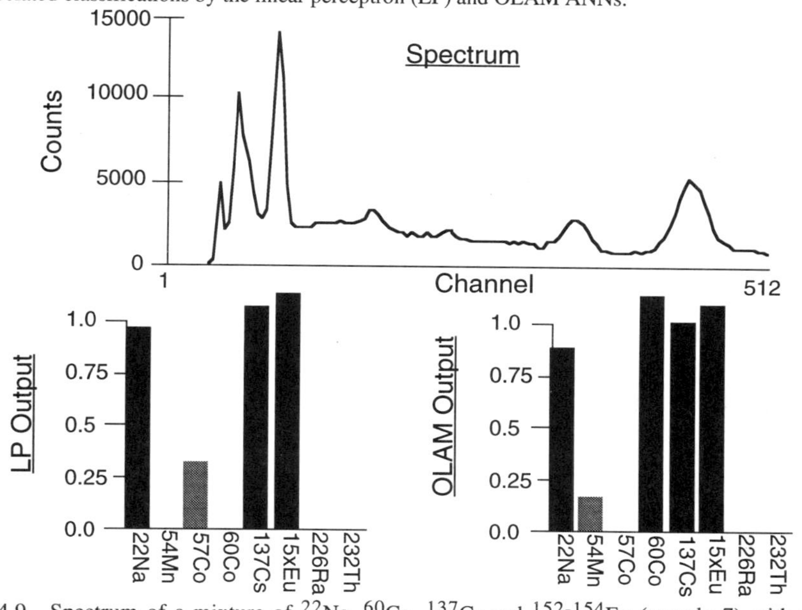

Figure 4.9. Spectrum of a mixture of ^{22}Na, ^{60}Co, ^{137}Cs and $^{152\text{-}154}Eu$ (sample 7) with the associated classifications by the linear perceptron (LP) and the OLAM ANNs. ANN outputs in gray indicate incorrect identification of an isotope.

Table 4.3: Classification of actual spectra from NaI detector with linear perceptron (LP) and OLAM. Each column represents a different isotope. RMS Error is listed in the right-hand column.

	^{22}Na	^{54}Mn	^{57}Co	^{60}Co	^{137}Cs	^{15x}Eu	^{226}Ra	^{232}Th	Error
Sample 1 (^{60}Co)									
Actual	0.00	0.00	0.00	1.00	0.00	0.00	0.00	0.00	
LP	0.01	0.08	0.00	1.00	0.00	0.00	0.00	0.07	0.038
OLAM	0.00	0.00	0.00	1.00	0.00	0.00	0.00	0.00	0.000
Sample 2 ($^{152\text{-}154}$Eu)									
Actual	0.00	0.00	0.00	0.00	0.00	1.00	0.00	0.00	
LP	0.00	0.00	0.00	0.00	0.00	1.00	0.00	0.00	0.000
OLAM	0.00	0.00	0.00	0.00	0.00	1.00	0.00	0.00	0.000
Sample 3 (^{226}Ra)									
Actual	0.00	0.00	0.00	0.00	0.00	0.00	1.00	0.00	
LP	0.00	0.00	0.00	0.01	0.00	0.00	1.00	0.00	0.004
OLAM	0.00	0.00	0.00	0.00	0.00	0.00	1.00	0.00	0.000
Sample 4 (Mixture of ^{60}Co and ^{137}Cs)									
Actual	0.00	0.00	0.00	1.00	1.00	0.00	0.00	0.00	
LP	0.06	0.00	0.27	0.62	1.01	0.02	0.01	0.00	0.166
OLAM	0.02	0.00	0.00	1.15	1.01	0.00	0.00	0.00	0.054
Sample 5 (Mixture of ^{22}Na, ^{57}Co, ^{60}Co, ^{137}Cs, and ^{15x}Eu)									
Actual	1.00	0.00	1.00	1.00	1.00	1.00	0.00	0.00	
LP	0.96	0.00	0.38	0.00	1.00	1.21	0.02	0.00	0.423
OLAM	0.85	0.00	0.67	1.41	1.00	1.17	0.00	0.00	0.203
Sample 6 (Mixture of ^{60}Co, ^{137}Cs, and ^{15x}Eu)									
Actual	0.00	0.00	0.00	1.00	1.00	1.00	0.00	0.00	
LP	0.08	0.00	0.40	0.00	0.95	1.13	0.03	0.00	0.385
OLAM	0.00	0.23	0.00	1.61	0.97	1.10	0.00	0.00	0.233
Sample 7 (Mixture of ^{22}Na, ^{60}Co, ^{137}Cs, and ^{15x}Eu)									
Actual	1.00	0.00	0.00	1.00	1.00	1.00	0.00	0.00	
LP	0.96	0.00	0.32	0.00	1.05	1.12	0.02	0.00	0.374
OLAM	0.86	0.18	0.00	1.32	1.04	1.09	0.00	0.00	0.143

Table 4.4: Classification of Monte-Carlo generated spectra simulating a NaI detector with linear perceptron (LP) and OLAM ANNs. Each column represents a different isotope. RMS Error is listed in the right-hand column.

	^{22}Na	^{54}Mn	^{57}Co	^{60}Co	^{137}Cs	^{15x}Eu	^{226}Ra	^{232}Th	Error
Sample 1 (Mixture of ^{60}Co and ^{137}Cs)									
Actual	0.00	0.00	0.00	1.00	1.00	0.00	0.00	0.00	
LP	0.00	0.00	0.00	0.89	0.72	0.00	0.00	0.00	0.106
OLAM	0.00	0.00	0.00	1.00	1.00	0.00	0.00	0.00	0.000
Sample 2 (Mixture of ^{22}Na, ^{54}Mn, ^{57}Co, ^{60}Co and ^{137}Cs)									
Actual	1.00	1.00	1.00	1.00	1.00	0.00	0.00	0.00	
LP	0.00	0.41	0.70	0.66	0.00	0.00	0.00	0.00	0.441
OLAM	1.00	1.00	1.00	1.00	1.00	0.00	0.00	0.00	0.000
Sample 3 (Mixture of 0.5 ^{22}Na, ^{57}Co, and 0.7 ^{137}Cs)									
Actual	0.50	0.00	1.00	0.00	0.70	0.00	0.00	0.00	
LP	0.00	0.00	0.90	0.00	0.15	0.00	0.00	0.00	0.350
OLAM	0.50	0.00	1.00	0.00	0.70	0.00	0.00	0.00	0.000
Sample 4 (^{54}Mn with peak reduced by 50%)									
Actual	0.00	0.50	0.00	0.00	0.00	0.00	0.00	0.00	
LP	0.00	0.49	0.00	0.00	0.00	0.00	0.00	0.00	0.004
OLAM	0.01	0.50	0.00	0.01	0.01	0.00	0.00	0.00	0.006
Sample 5 (^{54}Mn with only peak)									
Actual	0.00	1.00	0.00	0.00	0.00	0.00	0.00	0.00	
LP	0.00	1.01	0.00	0.00	0.00	0.00	0.00	0.00	0.004
OLAM	0.00	0.98	0.00	0.00	0.00	0.00	0.00	0.00	0.006

Results from the alpha spectral qualification study show that only integrated or low resolution data are required for inferring reasonable decisions about the quality of the data. The results indicate that the ANN based approach is ready for inclusion into an automatic system for assessing quality of alpha spectra. Because inference is possible with reduced resolution, the commonly limited resources of in-line process monitoring equipment should still accommodate the ANN approach. Both quality and isotope identification alarm systems appear feasible and practical.

Results from the isotope identification system have shown the superior performance of the OLAM approach over the linear perceptron for gamma-ray spectral analysis in both classification accuracy and training speed. The classification performance can be attributed to the orthogonalization process used by the OLAM during training. Since this training process is non-iterative, the OLAM offers a substantially shorter training time than the linear perceptron. Also, this system illustrates that isotopes in a contaminant can be identified in a fraction of a second once the spectrum is sent to the ANN.

One of the disadvantages of the OLAM is that nearly ideal spectra are needed in the training process. However, if needed, the OLAM can be provided with Monte Carlo generated spectra. The linear perceptron can be trained with noisy data or data with defects as long as a large training set is available.

Further work could involve comparison of the ANN approach to more conventional techniques, exploration of other ANN paradigms, examination of techniques for combining ANN models, and development of field prototype systems. A field deployable system should work with different source geometries and should compensate for pile-up and gain shifting. An ANN that handles gain-shifting was recently reported by Olmos *et. al.*.[16]

Information on ANN developments at Pacific Northwest National Laboratory is available in the World Wide Web (WWW) pages of the Environmental Molecular Sciences Laboratory which is accessible through such WWW clients as Netscape and NCSA Mosaic.

URL: http://www.emsl.pnl.gov:2080/docs/cie/neural/

4.9. Acknowledgments

The authors wish to thank Brian Keele of Westinghouse Hanford Company for graciously providing gamma-ray spectra for this study.

4.10. References

1. B.G. Levi, "Hanford seeks short- and long-term solutions to its legacy of waste," *Physics Today* **45(3)** (1992) 17-21.
2. D.L. Wanningman, R.R. Farrell, A.V. Rochini and G.L. Troyer, "Analysis of Alpha CAM Performance at the Waste Isolation Pilot Plant (WIPP)," in *Health Physics Society 39th Annual Meeting* (San Francisco, CA, 1994), paper WAM-F6.
3. G.L. Troyer, "Algorithms To Correct For Radon Progeny Interference," in *Health Physics Society 37th Annual Meeting*, paper WAM-E4, Columbus, OH, June 1992.
4. M.K. Alam, S.L. Stanton and G.A. Hebner, "Near-Infrared Spectroscopy and Neural Networks for Resin Identification," *Spectroscopy* **9(2)** (1994) 30-40.

5. J.M. Lerner and T. Lu, "Practical Neural Networks Aid Spectroscopic Analysis," *Photonic Spectra* (August 1993) 93-98.
6. H. Lohninger and F. Stancl, "Comparing the performance of neural networks to well-established methods of multivariate data analysis: the classification of mass spectral data," *Fresenius Journal of Analytical Chemistry* **344** (1992) 186-189.
7. B.J. Wythoff, S.P. Levine and S.A. Tomellini, "Spectral Peak Verification and Recognition Using a Multilayered Neural Network," *Analytical Chemistry* **60** (1990) 2702-2709.
8. D.E. Rumelhart, G.E. Hinton and R.J. Williams, "Learning Internal Representations by Error Propagation," in *Parallel Distributed Processing Systems*, (MIT Press, Cambridge, MA, 1986), vol. 1, pp. 318-362.
9. P. Olmos, J.C. Diaz, J.M. Perez, P. Gomez, V. Rodellar, P. Aguayo, A. Bru, G. Garcia-Belmonte and J.L. de Pablos, "A New Approach to Automatic Radiation Spectrum Analysis," *IEEE Transactions on Nuclear Science* **38** (1991) 971-975.
10. P. Olmos, J.C. Diaz, J.M. Perez, G. Garcia-Belmonte, P. Gomez and V. Rodellar, "Application of neural network techniques in gamma spectroscopy," *Nuclear Instruments and Methods in Physics Research* **A312** (1992) 167-173.
11. R. Koohi-Fayegh, S. Green, N.M.J. Crout, G.C. Taylor and M.C. Scott, "Neural network unfolding of photon and neutron spectra using an NE-213 scintillation detector," *Nuclear Instruments and Methods in Physics Research* **A329** (1993) 269-276.
12. P.E. Keller, R.T. Kouzes and L.J. Kangas, "Applications of Neural Networks to Real-Time Data Processing at the Environmental and Molecular Sciences Laboratory," in *Conference Record of the Eighth Conference on Real-Time Computer Applications in Nuclear, Particle and Plasma Physics*, (TRIUMF, Vancouver, BC, Canada, 1993), pp. 438-440.
13. F. Rosenblatt, "Two theorems of statistical separability in the Perceptron," in *Mechanisation of Thought Process, Proceedings of symposium No. 10,* (National Physical Laboratory, London, 1958), vol. I, pp. 421-456.
14. T. Kohonen, "Correlation matrix memories," *IEEE Transactions on Computers* **C-21** (1972) 353.
15. T. Kohonen, *Self Organization and Associative Memory*, third ed., (Springer-Verlag, New York, 1989).
16. P. Olmos, J.C. Diaz, J.M. Perez, P. Aguayo, P. Gomez, and V. Rodellar, "Drift Problems in the Automatic Analysis of Gamma-Ray Spectra Using Associative Memory Algorithms," *IEEE Transactions on Nuclear Science* **41** (1994) 637-641.

5. NEURAL NETWORK UTILITY IN NONDESTRUCTIVE TRANSURANIC WASTE ASSAY, INITIAL INVESTIGATIONS

GREG BECKER
Idaho National Engineering Laboratory†, *Lockheed Idaho Technologies Company,*
P.O. Box 1625, MS 2114
Idaho Falls, Idaho 83145, USA
E-mail: gkb1@inel.gov

ABSTRACT

The determination of transuranic (TRU) and associated radioactive material quantities entrained in waste forms is a necessary component of waste characterization. Measurement performance requirements are specified in the National TRU Waste Characterization Program quality assurance plan for which compliance must be demonstrated prior to the transportation and disposition of wastes. With respect to this criterion, the existing TRU nondestructive waste assay (NDA) capability is inadequate for a significant fraction of the U.S Department of Energy (DOE) complex waste inventory. This is a result of the general application of safeguard-type measurement and calibration schemes to waste form configurations. Incompatibilities between such measurement methods and actual waste form configurations complicate regulation compliance demonstration processes and illustrate the need for an alternate measurement interpretation paradigm.

Hence, it appears necessary to supplement or perhaps restructure the perceived solution and approach to the waste NDA problem. The first step is to understand the magnitude of the waste matrix/source attribute space associated with those waste form configurations in inventory and how this creates complexities and unknowns with respect to existing NDA methods. Once defined and/or bounded, a conceptual method must be developed that specifies the necessary tools and the framework in which the tools are used. A promising framework is a hybridized neural network structure. Discussed are some typical complications associated with conventional waste NDA techniques and how improvements can be obtained through the application of neural networks.

5.1. Overview

Techniques commonly utilized to acquire nondestructive assay data on TRU waste forms are for the most part based on gamma and/or neutron-type measurements. The investigations undertaken in this work concern the performance of neural networks with respect to the passive neutron measurement technique. A

---

†This work was supported by the U.S. Department of Energy (DOE), Assistant Secretary for Environmental Management, under DOE Idaho Operations Office Contract DE-AC07-94ID13223.

comparison of the neural network based system relative to the conventional passive/active neutron system commonly employed at many DOE sites is then made.

Prior to a discussion of the procedure and results, it is necessary to understand those waste NDA issues that have prompted investigations into alternate methods. This is best accomplished via an overview of the waste form configurations followed by a discussion of the capability of existing waste NDA systems and methods. The DOE TRU 208-L waste form inventory spans an enormous n-dimensional space in terms of matrix and source configurations influencing conventional NDA system response. For the moment, container sizes other than the 208-L drum are ignored. Attributes of such configurations can be categorized in terms of the waste matrix, the entrained radioactive material composition (TRU and non-TRU), and characteristics resulting from the combination of the previous two categories.

Waste matrix parameters that affect the response of an NDA system include the elemental composition, the volume averaged density, and element specific density distributions in space. Characteristics of the entrained radioactive material affecting system response include the radionuclidic/isotopic composition, the radioactive material chemical compound and/or mixture, the spatial distribution of the radioactive material, and the density distribution of the radioactive material, e.g., diffuse, aggregate, unit pieces or a combination thereof. One then must understand the interaction between these two parameters, which further convolutes the measurement task. Such interactions include gamma attenuation, nuclear reactions (α,n), neutron moderation/absorption, etc.

It is next instructive to look at the functional aspects of the commonly employed passive/active neutron type system used for waste NDA of 208-L drums. The passive/active neutron system operates in two modes: a passive neutron coincidence counting mode and an active neutron interrogation mode. Response data acquired via these two measurements are used as appropriate to arrive at a mass value for TRU material entrained within a given 208-L (55-gal) drum waste container. The active mode is confined to the lower mass range, less than a few grams of fissile material, and the passive is employed above this. The two modes are not entirely independent as some minor response corrections derived from one mode are applied to the other.

The passive/active neutron system is calibrated to quantify the mass of specific isotopes associated with the source composition associated with a given inventory population. This implies that in a stand-alone operational mode, the source composition must be *a priori* known. The source composition used for measurement purposes in this study is one which comprises a significant fraction of the DOE inventory, weapons grade plutonium (WG Pu). For this composition, the passive neutron mode signal comes from the ^{240}Pu isotope, and in the active mode, it is due to ^{239}Pu. The balance of radionuclides associated with the WG Pu, e.g. ^{241}Am, can be established in terms of relative mass ratios with respect to the quantified ^{240}Pu and ^{239}Pu isotopes, provided a means is available such as high-resolution gamma spectroscopy. This is one method whereby a measure of the total mass and associated quantities, alpha activity, thermal power, etc., can be acquired.

This NDA measurement approach works reasonably well and, in general, complies with applicable National TRU Waste Characterization Program quality assurance objectives when *the waste form is compatible with the response characteristics and capability of the system.* In other words, the design of the passive/active neutron instrument as well as the calibration scheme employed is based on a conceptual understanding of the physical properties of the DOE complex waste form inventory. The performance and capability of the instrument are a function of the degree of agreement between the actual waste form and the instrument design/calibration concept.

Certainly, it is not possible to devise a simple measurement scheme based on a single modality, neutron (supplemented by high resolution γ spectroscopy), which can accommodate the myriad of waste form configurations throughout the complex, let alone a subpopulation residing at a single site. Indeed, experience has shown that the passive/active neutron system capabilities are confined to a definite waste matrix/source configuration realm. For example, the performance of the passive neutron coincidence-counting technique employed in this type of system is sufficient if the moderating properties and density of the matrix are within certain values. Additionally, this technique works well if the source isotopic and chemical composition does not produce an (α,n) neutron component of sufficient magnitude to interfere with the coincidence-counting technique. Unfortunately, actual waste forms are comprised of matrix and source configurations that strongly interfere with the passive neutron technique. Additional and, in fact, more serious interferences are associated with the active mode of the neutron system. The high-resolution gamma spectroscopy system is also subject to complications arising from commonly encountered matrix/source configurations.

This is not to say every waste container exhibits matrix/source properties that confound the measurement system. There are several matrix/source configurations that do not possess inherently complicating characteristics allowing the acquisition of meaningful data. This is fine, but the result of this situation is to force one into the less desirable situation of attempting to define what waste forms the measurement system can handle and those it cannot. Thus, we no longer have a viable waste NDA capability, but rather a system with specific functional boundaries that require significant resources to establish and maintain. Even with this type of method in place, an on-line method of determining which waste containers are within the system capability and which must be returned to storage is necessary. Depending on the waste form, the proportion of drums that are returned to storage can be significant.

In summary the general state of waste NDA capability as it exists today is inadequate. National TRU Waste Program requirements dictate a 100% completeness criterium, i.e., assay data are required for all waste containers. As it is presently an undeniable fact that there are many waste forms for which valid assays cannot be acquired or be demonstrated to comply with applicable quality assurance objectives, alternative methods programs must be pursued.

5.2. Application/Method

The waste NDA technique used to generate response data for the neural network utility investigations is the passive neutron coincidence-counting technique. Measurement data are acquired by inserting the waste container, a 208-L drum in this study, into the counting chamber and passively recording neutron events. To allow for an evaluation of neural network passive neutron data interpretation performance, the response of a passive/active waste NDA system commonly employed at DOE sites is used as a baseline. Measurement data are recorded simultaneously in both systems by simply extracting neutron event signals from the passive/active neutron system and routing them to a separate coincidence counting system used as the data source for the neural network training and testing. Therefore, the measurement apparatus/detector front-end signal processing chain is identical, providing for a convenient means of system performance comparison.

In order to make a meaningful evaluation of the neural network capability, it is necessary to define the realm or n-dimensional space that the measurement sets encompass. This is accomplished by simplifying the response through the elimination of complications arising from matrix interactions. Thus, the first measurement set is acquired on an empty 208-L drum where only the position, mass, and neutronics of the drum are varied. Approximately 80 separate measurements were made for differing configurations of source spatial location, mass values, and source density distributions. Two-thirds of this data set were used for training with the balance serving as a test set. The measurement range in terms of source spatial distribution is determined by the internal dimensions of the drum. The mass of WG Pu associated with the data set ranged from 22 to 160 g. Neutronic effects were introduced primarily through source orientation and source volume density or proximity variations.

In addition to the empty drum measurement set, a number of acquisitions were performed using a simulated waste matrix. This matrix is comprised of hundreds of borosilicate glass vials, 5 cm^3 each, loaded into a number of 1-gal polyethylene bottles. A total of 20 such glass vial/polyethylene bottles are fitted into the 208-L drum, providing an accurate representation of a common TRU waste form. In a manner similar to the empty drum measurement series, a number of measurements were made on the glass vial/polyethylene bottle matrix drum by varying source mass (20 to 260 g), position, and the neutronics.

5.3. Experimental Results

A backpropagation neural network was trained on the empty drum measurement series data. As expected, the nonlinearity and complexity of the system required a network with two hidden layers. The network did train after about 80 epochs, which indicates that the network architecture is appropriate for this problem. The training and test set data as processed through the network are illustrated in Figure 5.1, expressed as a relative percent difference between the neural network derived ^{240}Pu mass value and the actual ^{240}Pu mass value ratioed to the actual ^{240}Pu mass, the quantity of interest.

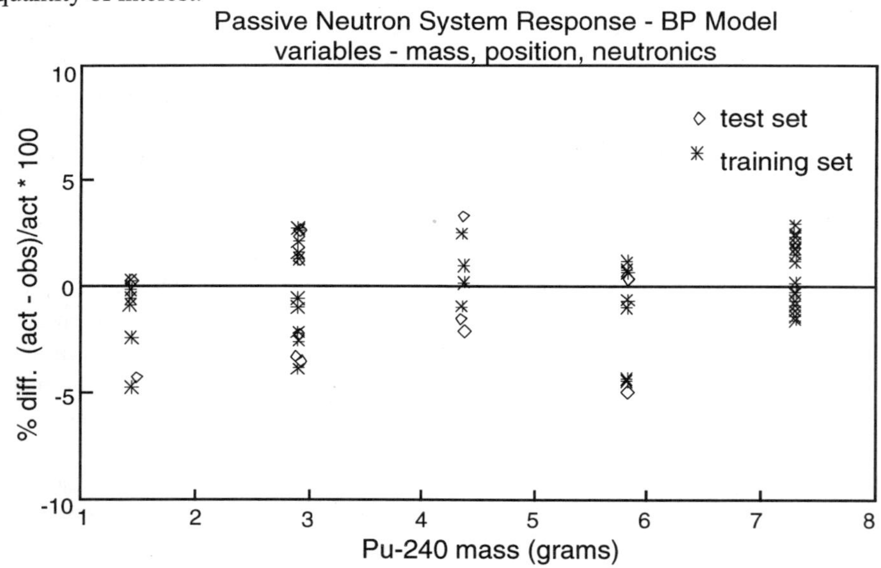

Figure 5.1. Empty drum back propagation model performance.

Evident are reasonable deviations from the true value despite the range of variations through source mass, position, and neutronics. The largest percent deviation is less than ±5% as compared to the response of the conventional passive/active system variation of ±30%. Such an improvement is significant as it represents the capability to decrease measurement uncertainty components by a magnitude useful in the compliance demonstration process. It also depicts the neural network capacity to quickly capture a complex phenomena without employing laborious analytical methods. In fact, the existing conventional system is such an analytical technique derived through a calibration routine.

The glass vial/polyethylene bottle data set was trained using a network with two hidden layers and also converged relatively quick. The largest percent deviation is slightly greater than ±5% as compared to the response of the conventional passive/active system variation of ±35%. The relative percent difference ratios are shown in Figure 5.2. Due to the paucity of measurement data, only the training data are shown. Nevertheless, it is evident that the network can and does embody the complex interaction of the matrix and source variations that are embedded in the system response.

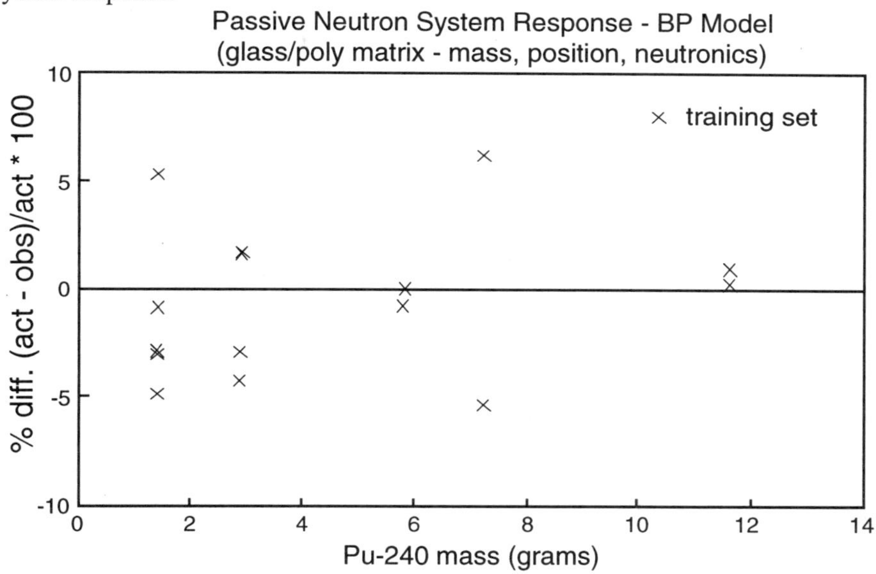

Figure 5.2. Glass vial/polyethylene vial neural network performance.

A third network was trained simply to yield information regarding the realm of applicability of a given network. For example, how well can a network trained for the empty drum and glass vial/polyethylene case perform if a similar network architecture is employed. The results of combining the measurement sets associated with these two measurement configurations is shown in Figure 5.3. It is clear that the performance of such a network is not as good as the networks trained on either the empty or glass vial/polyethylene matrix separately. This indicates that there is additional complexity introduced into the model that cannot be managed by the architectures used for either the empty drum or glass/polyethylene networks. Certainly, a network architecture could be devised to suit the combined glass polyethylene data. The important point is that the performance of the trained network is domain specific.

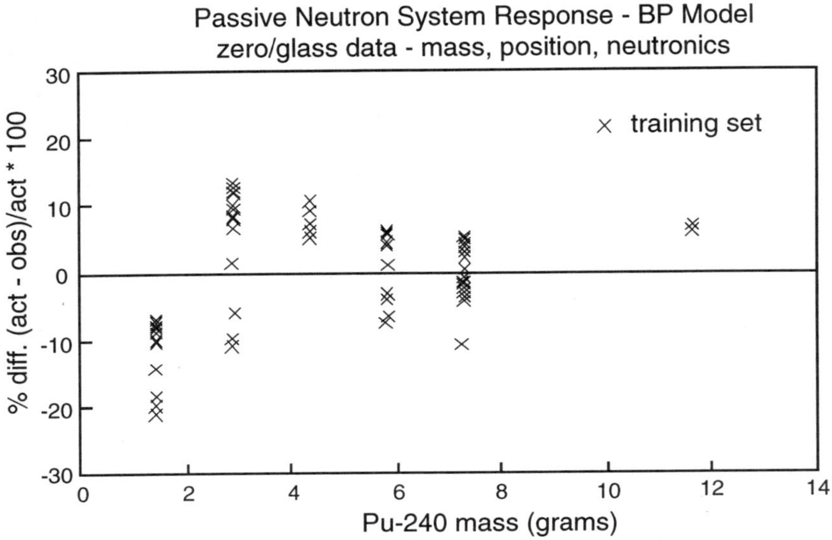

Figure 5.3. Combined empty drum and glass vial/polyethylene with inappropriate network architecture.

5.4. Conclusions

It is clear that the neural network tool is applicable to the complex waste NDA problem. The successful adaptation of such a method is strongly dependent on ensuring that the waste container to be assayed for its TRU content is within the realm of the network capacity. As indicated, the indiscriminate use of a network trained for one waste form attribute set or configuration applied to another yields less-than-desirable results. Future work will concern mechanisms to preprocess and categorize waste form populations such that characteristics associated with a given waste container can be identified as a member of a predefined category for which the response space is bounded. At this point, it is a straightforward procedure to process the data yielding those parameters of interest. It is exceedingly important that such a system have an inherent means to ensure that non-unique containers are not falsely categorized with a pre-specified degree of confidence.

6. APPLICATION OF NEURAL NETWORKS TO DETERMINE MOISTURE CONTENT ON HUMIDITY-ATTENUATED NEAR INFRARED (NIR) SPECTRA

TOMAS LOPEZ
Westinghouse Hanford Company†, P.O. Box 1970, MS L5-55
Richland, Washington 99352, USA
E-mail: tomas_lopez@rl.gov

BARBARA L. PHILIPP
ICF Kaiser, P.O. Box 1970, MS E6-21
Richland, Washington 99352, USA
E-mail: barbara_l_philipp@rl.gov

and

S. THOMPSON-BACHMEIER
Department of Electrical Engineering, Washington State University
Pullman, Washington 99164-2752, USA

ABSTRACT

Moisture has been identified as one of the critical tank waste parameters that impacts the safety status of the wastes, particularly tanks containing ferro/ferricyanide materials. Since water content is affected by a number of factors, including gravity, one hypothesis, currently being tested by Westinghouse Hanford's Waste Tank Safety organization, is that the surface of the waste contains a minimum of water compared to the material deeper in the tank. Assuming this hypothesis is correct, a minimum internal waste water content will be obtained by measuring the surface water content. Near infrared analysis is a nondestructive technique that takes advantage of the tendency of water molecules to absorb specific wavelengths of NIR energy. When a sample containing water is exposed to those wavelengths, a certain portion of the energy will be absorbed by the water, and the remainder will be reflected. By measuring the reflected energy, the concentration of water in the sample can be determined.

An initial investigation into the feasibility of remote sensing for hot cell and waste tank applications was performed at the University of Washington's Center for Process Analytical Chemistry (CPAC) under the direction of Westinghouse Hanford Company. The BY-104 waste tank simulant test data showed that for these samples, ten percent of the incident radiation is scattered. When collected, this signal is available for determining moisture content because the moisture content of the waste affects the scattering. However, atmospheric relative humid-

---

†This work was sponsored by the U.S. Department of Energy, EM-50 Program Office. Westinghouse Hanford Company is the Hanford Operations Contractor for the U.S. Department of Energy under Contract DE-AC06-87RL10930.

ity causes a signal attenuation that will impact any *in situ* measurements being obtained.

For simulation, this spectra was used along with software generated atmospheric transmission data from 0-60 meters to produce a modified sample set. These data are analyzed using a backpropagation neural network algorithm to construct a model that would predict surface moisture content. Predicted results are compared to moisture values generated using a Partial Least Squares algorithm.

6.1. Data Set

Table 6.1: In-Situ Waste Tank Environment

	In-Tank Physical Data
Temperature:	65° - 190°F
Pressure:	-2.5” to +1” H_20 (measured in head space)
Radiation Flux:	75 - 900 R/hr (in head space)
• Radiation:	Up to $10.5x10^3$ R/hr (gamma and beta) within waste
• Gamma:	less than $2.0x10^3$ R/hr
Relative Humidity:	10 percent - 100 percent (head space)
Moisture Content:	> 20 percent for solid waste
Specific Gravity:	1.2 to 2.0 for solid or liquid waste
Corrosivity:	Condensed vapors - pH from 8 to 14
	liquids - pH from 8 to 14, up to 3.56M NaOH
	solids - pH from 8 to 14 and up to 3.56M NaOH
Hazardous Location:	Class 1, Division 1, Group B per NEC Article 500

Table 6.2: Tank 241-BY-104 Modified Simulant Recipe

Compound	**Formula**	**Weight%**
sodium nitrate	$NaNO_3$	81.8%
sodium aluminate	$NaAlO_2$	7.5%
sodium hydroxide	NaOH	1.7%
sodium metasilicate	Na_2SiO_3	1.5%
ferric nitrate	$Fe(NO_3)_3$	1.0 %
sodium phosphate	Na_3PO_4	0.7%
calcium nitrate	$Ca(NO_3)_2$	0.4%
magnesium nitrate	$Mg(NO_3)_2$	0.2%
manganese (II) nitrate	$Mn(NO_3)_2$	0.2%
water	H_2O	5-25%

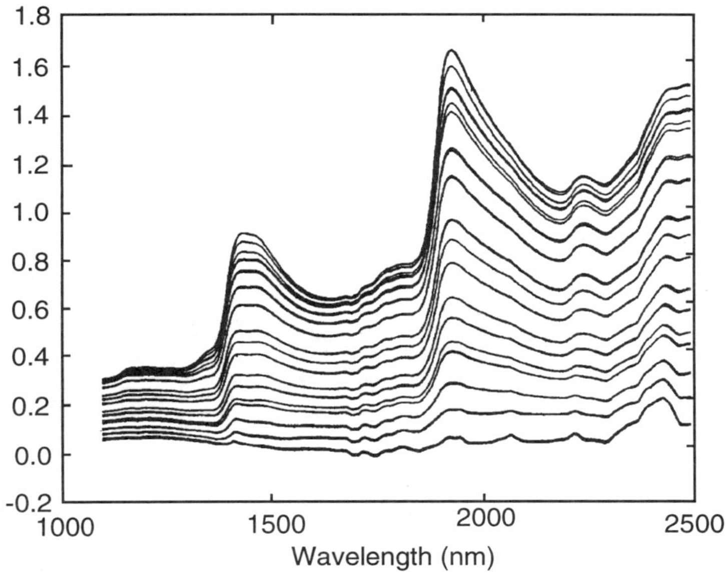

Figure 6.1. Near infrared (NIR) data set from CPAC task #1.

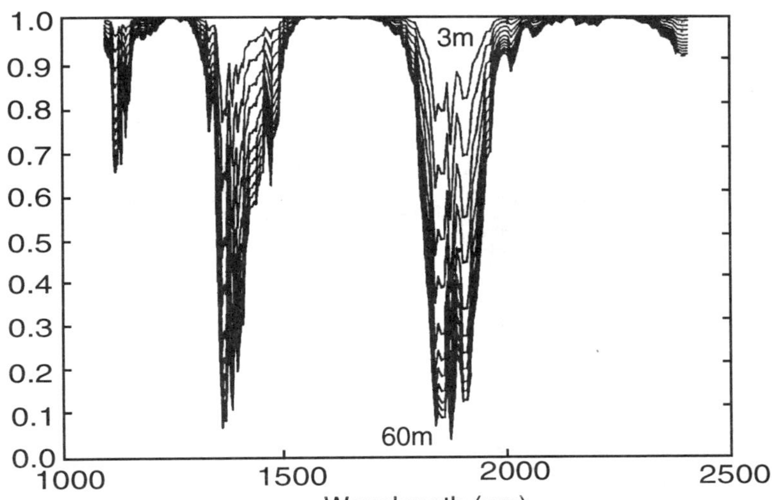

Figure 6.2. Atmospheric signal losses at 80% relative humidity over distances of 0 to 60 meters as modeled by LOWTRAN.

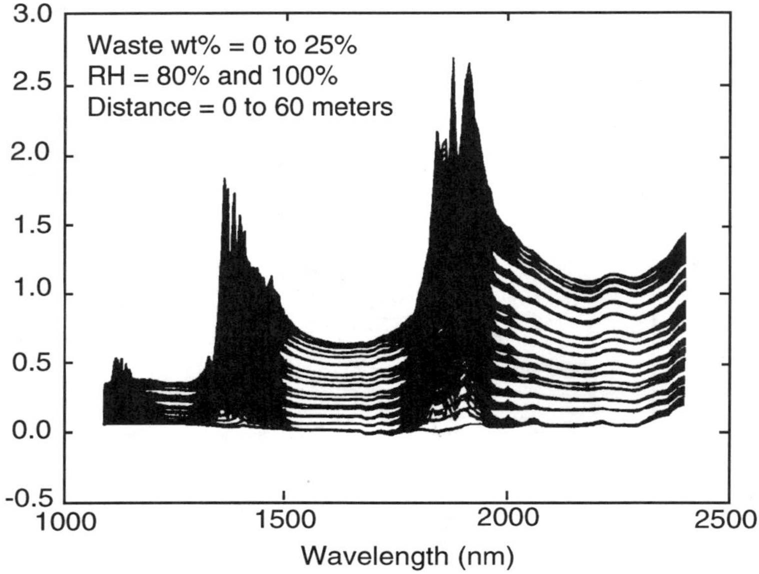

Figure 6.3. Apparent absorbance over distances of 0 to 60 meters.

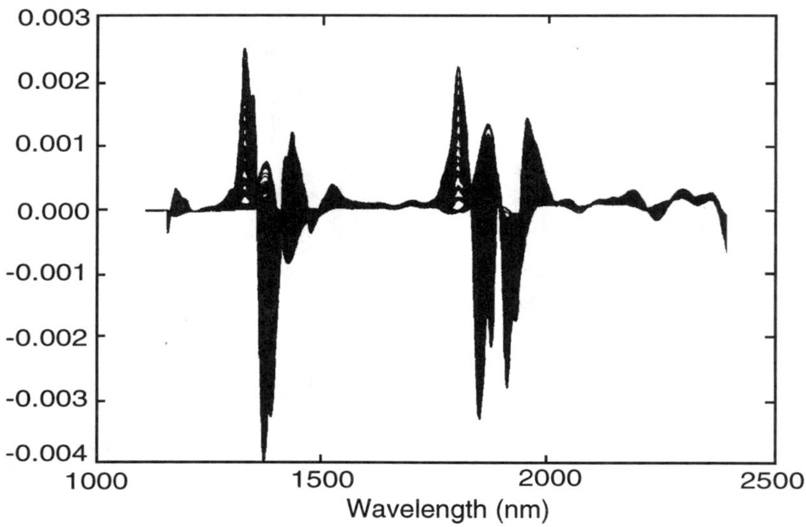

Figure 6.4. 2nd derivative of CPAC data including relative humidity transmission effects.

There are 900 total samples. Each set number contains 25 spectra for a total of 36 sets. The complete data set was split in half so there were 450 samples for training and 450 samples for testing. Alternating spectra were used for training and testing (i.e., Spectra #1 = Training, Spectra #2 = Testing, Spectra #3 = Training, etc.). Table 6.3 lists the concentrations for each set number.

Table 6.3: Moisture concentrations for each set (a set contains 25 spectra)

Set Number	Concentration	Set Number	Concentration
1 2 3 4	0.000	19 20	9.624
5 6	0.730	21 22	10.806
7 8	1.192	23 24	13.328
9 10	2.792	25 26	15.000
11 12	3.585	27 28	17.028
13 14	5.105	29 30	18.529
15 16	6.502	31 32	20.225
17 18	8.411	33 34	22.393
		35 36	25.820

Table 6.4: Each spectrum within each set is modified by humidity and distance effects (i.e. Set #1 (0%)).

Spectrum Number	Relative Humidity (%)	Distance (m)
1	Original Spectrum	
2	80	0
3	80	1
4	80	3
5	80	7
6	80	12
7	80	20
8	80	27
9	80	33
10	80	40
11	80	47
12	80	53
13	80	60
14	100	0
15...	...	...

6.2. Neural Network Model

6.2.1. Network Design

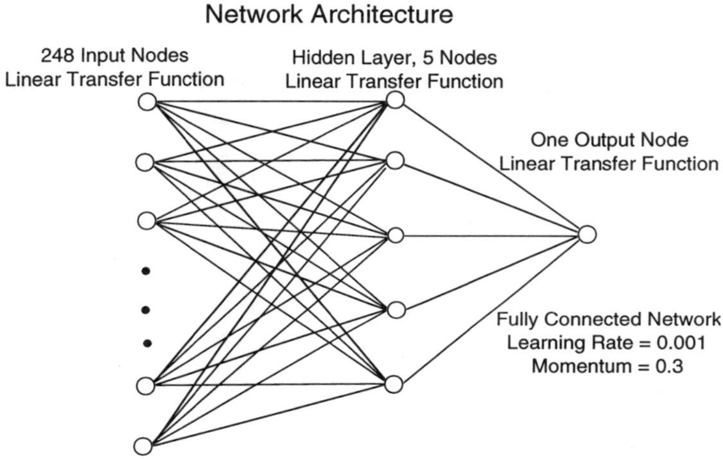

Figure 6.5. Network architecture of neural network used to predict moisture content.

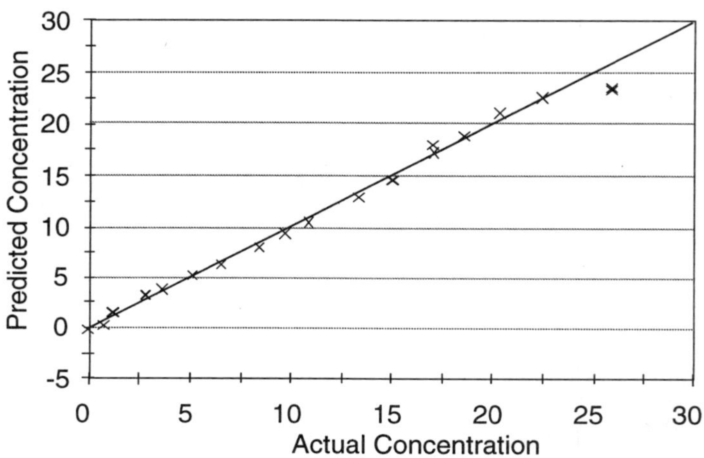

Figure 6.6. Plot of the actual concentration versus the neural network predicted concentration.

6.2.2. Network Performance: Noise Effects

How does a network trained on noiseless data respond to noisy data? How does a network trained on noisy data respond to noisy data? Results of the noise tests are listed in Table 6.5 and plotted in Figure 6.7.

Table 6.5: Results of Noise Tests

Training Conditions	Testing Conditions	Results	
		Avg. Error	Std. Dev.
w/o Noise	w/o Noise	-0.182	0.677
	S/N=1	-5.115	73.108
	S/N=10	0.293	7.484
	S/N=100	-0.154	0.963
	S/N=1000	-0.183	0.681
S/N= 100	w/o Noise	-0.125	0.608
	S/N=1	1.501	43.450
	S/N=10	-0.117	4.339
	S/N=100	-0.139	0.742
	S/N=1000	-0.123	0.609

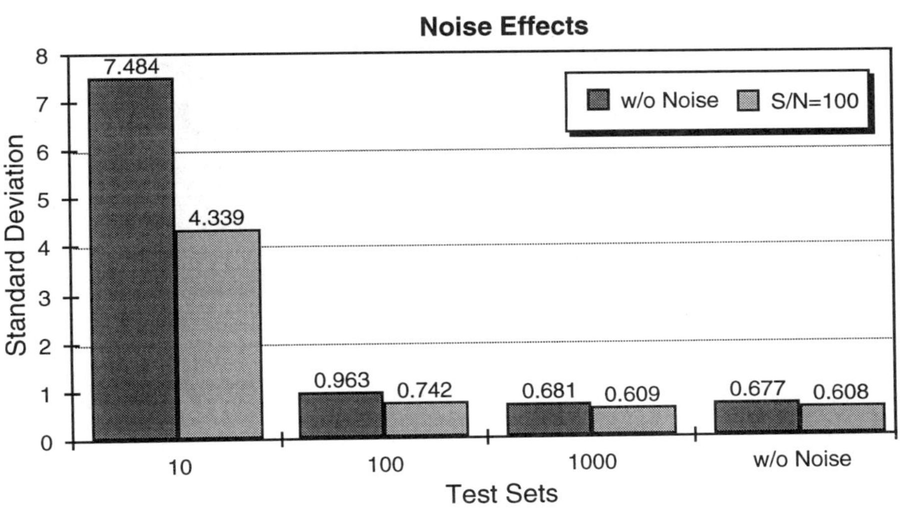

Figure 6.7. Results of noise tests.

6.2.3. Network Performance: Interpolation Effects

How does a network respond to a spectral concentration it has not been trained on? Results of the interpolation tests are listed in Table 6.6 and plotted in Figure 6.8.

Table 6.6: Results of Interpolation Tests

Training Conditions	Testing Conditions	Results	
		Avg. Error	Std. Error
All Spectra	All Spectra	-0.182	0.677
w/o 0.73%	0.73%	-0.342	0.088
	All Spectra	0.020	0.665
w/o 22.393%	22.393%	0.473	0.040
	All Spectra	-0.007	0.670

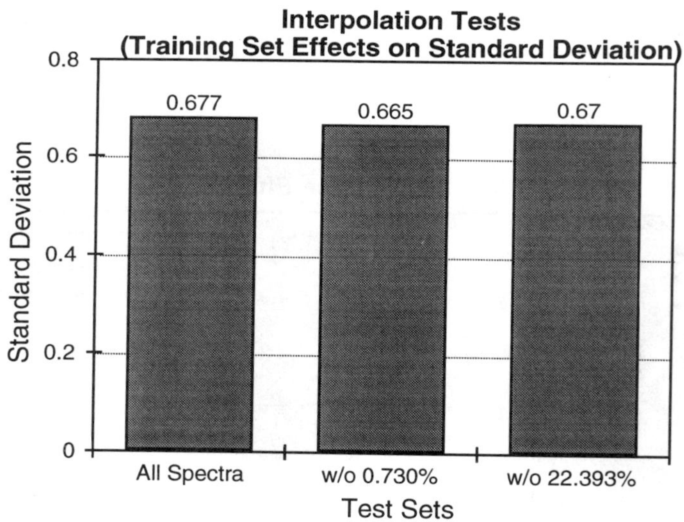

Figure 6.8. Results of interpolation tests.

6.2.4. Network Performance: Wavelength Shift

How does a network respond to shifted data? How does a network trained on shifted data respond to shifted data it has not been trained on? Results of the wavelength shift tests are listed in Table 6.7 and plotted in Figure 6.9.

Table 6.7: Results of Wavelength Shift Tests

Training Conditions	**Testing Conditions**	**Results**	
		Avg. Error	Std. Error
w/o Shift	0.0 nm	-0.182	0.677
	0.25 nm	0.428	0.794
	0.50 nm	1.039	1.073
	1.0 nm	2.260	1.800
w/ 0.25 nm, 0.50 nm,	0.0 nm	0.042	0.666
1.0 nm Shift	0.75 nm	0.009	0.675

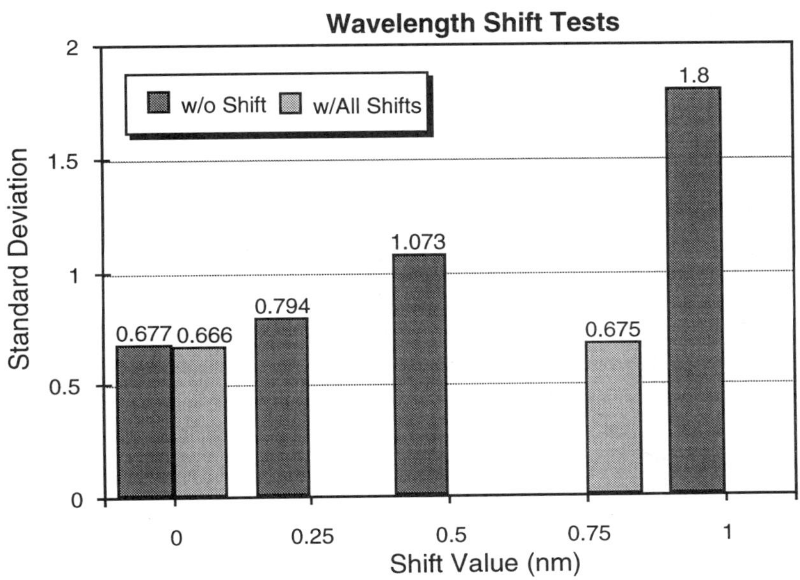

Figure 6.9. Results of wavelength shift tests.

6.3. Partial Least Squares (PLS) Model

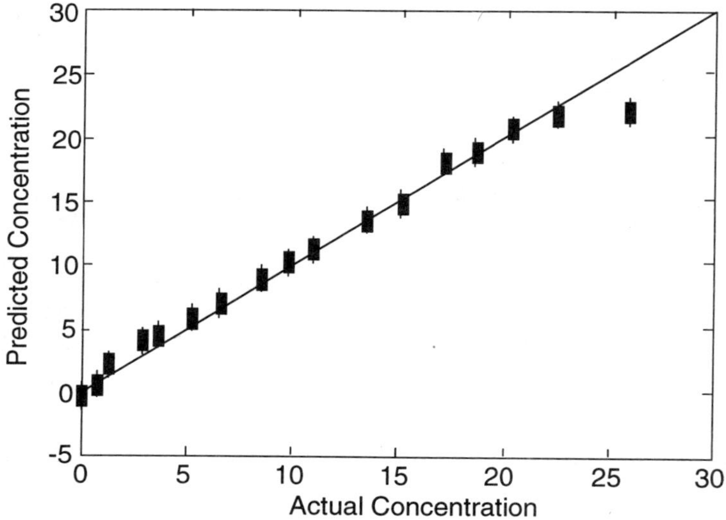

Figure 6.10. 2-factor partial least squares derivative data model. 2nd derivative CPAC task 1 data with 80% and 100% relative humidity data.

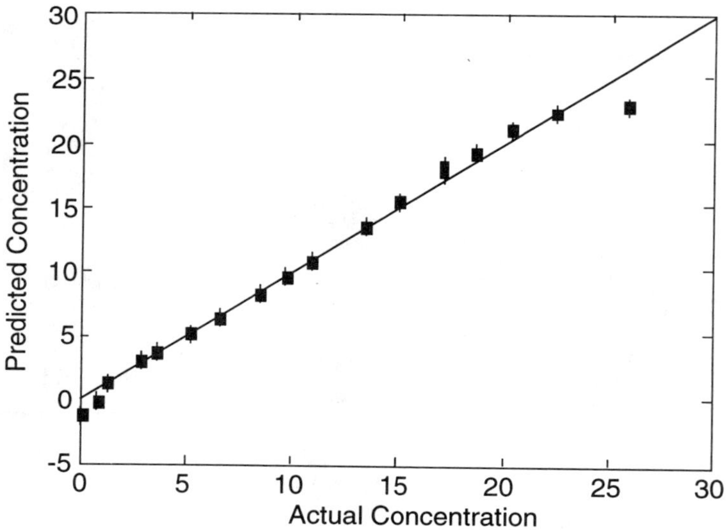

Figure 6.11. 3-factor partial least squares raw data model. CPAC task 1 data with 80% and 100% relative humidity data.

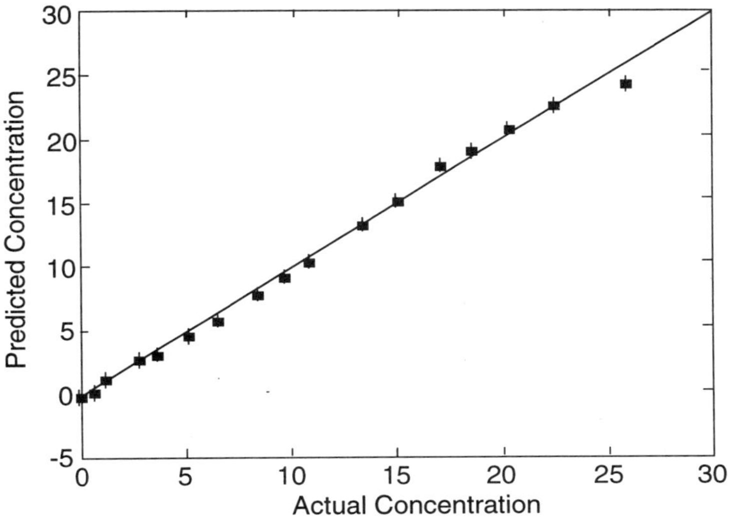

Figure 6.12. 3-factor partial least squares derivative data model. 2nd derivative CPAC task 1 data with 80% and 100% relative humidity data.

6.4. Conclusions

1) A Neural Network algorithm was shown to accurately predict moisture content of humidity-modified NIR spectra.
2) The model was tested to determine the effect of "real-world" impracticalities of the data (i.e., Noisy Data, Interpolation, X-Axis Shift).
   - Using a Noisy Training Set Improved the Network's Ability to Predict Moisture
   - The Network was able to Predict Unknown Concentrations Accurately.
   - Once Trained on Wavelength Shift, the Network was able to Accurately Predict Moisture on Untrained Shifts.
3) Future Work:
   - Investigate Non-Linear Effects at Higher Moisture Concentrations (>24%).
   - Investigate the Use of Derivative Data.

7. FLUORESCENT DIAGNOSTICS OF ORGANIC POLLUTION IN NATURAL WATERS: A NEURAL NETWORK APPROACH

YURI V. ORLOV, I.G. PERSIANTSEV, S.P. REBRIK
Microelectronics Department, Nuclear Physics Institute, Moscow State University
Moscow 119899, Russia
E-mail: orlov@neuro.npi.msu.su

and

SERGEY M. BABICHENKO
Institute of Ecology, Tallinn, Estonia

ABSTRACT

Rapid diagnosis of pollution is one of the key tasks in the field of ecological monitoring of natural and technogeneous environment. One of the promising methods of fluorescent diagnosis of organic pollution of water environment is the registration and analysis of two-dimensional Spectral Fluorescent Signatures (SFS).

The neural networks - based system suggested in this paper is intended for solving the problem of detection, identification, and concentration measurement of water environmental pollution. The suggested system uses SFS as input pattern and allows one to build a rapid diagnosis system for ecological monitoring.

7.1. Method of Spectral Signatures

In the SFS method,[1] the natural water is treated as an integral spectroscopic sample and is characterized by a certain specific two-dimensional SFS-spectrum, which is a matrix of emission intensity recorded in coordinates of excitation and emission wavelengths. For the fluorescent diagnostics of organic pollution an excitation range of 240-360 nm was used, and the spectral response was registered in the 200 nm wide window, red-shifted by 10 nm against the excitation wavelength. The standard size of the intensity matrix was 25 x 40 elements.

The analysis of SFS is hampered by the following:[2]

(a) camouflaging of the pollutant spectrum by the Dissolved Organic Matter (DOM) spectrum which depends on the season and on the geographical location (Figure 7.1);

(b) the dependence of the SFS shape on concentrations of the pollutant and DOM.

These reasons make it difficult to build a fixed set of all possible reference spectra that are necessary for classification by traditional methods (e.g. "nearest neighbor" method). The presence of the camouflaging spectrum decreases the reliability of analysis at low pollutant concentrations, i.e. in the most important cases.

The ability of a neural net to learn by examples and to generalize received information makes its use in this case very attractive.

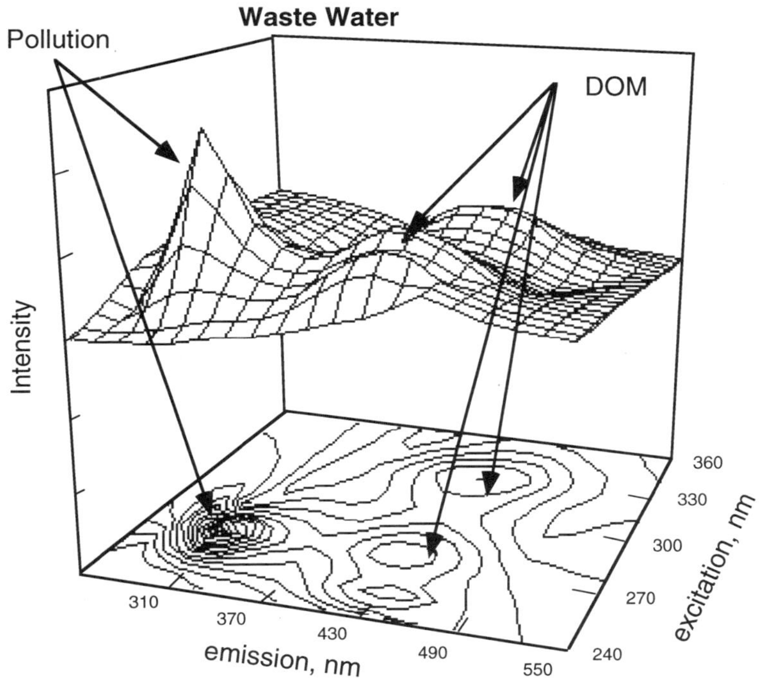

Figure 7.1. Typical SFS of a highly polluted waste water (DOM - Dissolved Organic Matter).

7.2. Training Procedure of the Neural Net

Our catalogue of potential water pollutants at the moment consists of more than 70 samples, including crude oils, diesel oils, light oil fractions, technical oils, residual oils and different phenols (reference spectra of solutions and emulsions of pollutants in bidistilled water).

The catalogue of spectral signatures of DOM for different aquatoria at present includes more than 15 samples mainly from the Baltic and the North Seas.

As recording conditions preclude saturation of the detector, and there is no chemical interaction between DOM, water, and the pollutant, the resulting spectrum appears to be a linear combination of three components: Raman Scattering Signal (RSS) of water molecules (Figure 7.2), fluorescence of DOM and fluorescence of the pollutant. The components' ratio in the spectrum depends on the concentration and fluorescence efficiency of the pollutant and DOM.

This allowed to synthesize the training spectrum for any given concentration of the pollutant just before presenting spectrum to the NN. To make the NN insensitive to variations of DOM spectra, different types of DOM spectra were used. All spectra were normalized to unity at the point of maximum intensity.

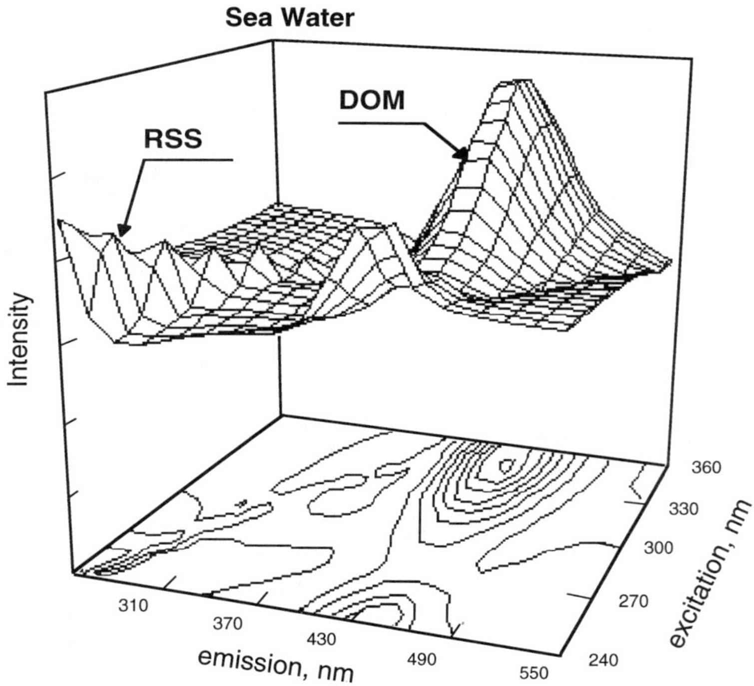

Figure 7.2. Typical SFS of sea water (RSS - Raman Scattering Signal from water molecules, DOM - Dissolved Organic Matter).

All NNs used in the suggested system are multi-layer perceptrons[3] trained by error back-propagation.[4] Training is based on the method of gradual complication of the task:[5] first, NN is trained to classify mixtures containing pollutants at high concentration, then, concentration of pollutants in the presented mixtures is gradually decreased. The training proceeds while the NN is able to maintain its performance at the acceptable level.

7.3. System Description

Depending on the amount of DOM concentration, one may distinguish two extreme cases of utilization of ecological monitoring system:

(a) at low DOM concentrations (e.g. during monitoring of open sea areas) the system should detect very low or trace concentrations of a pollutant (Figure 7.3);

(b) at high DOM concentrations that correspond, as a rule, to the situations of moderately or highly polluted waters (e.g. at initial stages of sewage treatment) the system should determine pollution components (presented generally at relatively high concentrations) as well as to detect dangerously high DOM concentrations.

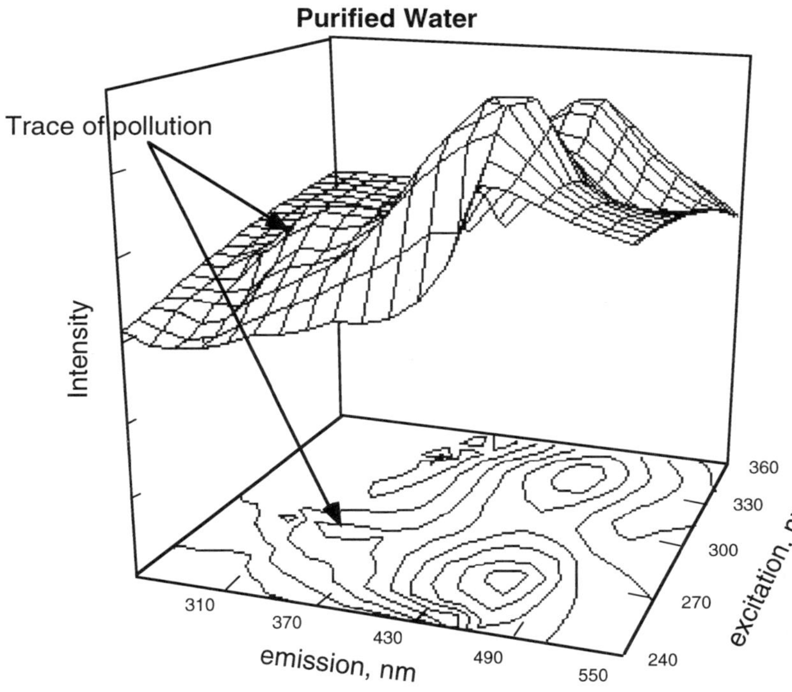

Figure 7.3. Typical SFS of purified water with slight trace of pollution.

In both of the above cases, the suggested system can work in either of the three modes:

1. It can detect "stress" conditions of the environment, namely, detect that technogeneous pollution exceeds a predetermined level. Such mode is sufficient for some applications, e.g. for monitoring of pollution accumulation in the areas of intensive navigation. In this case the system gives a qualitative answer (yes/no) and exact pollutant classification is not required.

2. The system can identify the pollutant(s) and measure it's concentration. In this case pollution classification is performed on the basis of end-user library of possible pollutants. A multistage procedure was elaborated for solving this task previously.[6] After rough classification into broad classes, pollutant identification within a previously determined class is made by a NN corresponding to the given class. Finally, concentration of the pollutant is determined by a linear NN corresponding to the identified pollutant. For this procedure a set of NNs arranged in a hierarchical tree-like structure can be used.
3. The system can perform pollution classification on the basis of "generalized" classes of pollutants. Our investigations show that all possible important technogeneous pollutants may be divided into 4 "generalized" classes: phenols, light oil products, medium oil products, and lubricants (Figure 7.4). This classification is based on the analysis of the spectral features of wide range of pollutants and is in good correlation with the pollutant's physical and chemical properties. Treating every pollutant in terms of "generalized" classes allows one to create rather universal system, thus widening the area of possible applications and increasing the number of potential users. On the other hand, identification of a pollutant is not possible in this case. Also, it should be noted that fluorescence efficiency of pollutants within a given "generalized" class may differ significantly. It means, that the accuracy of determination of concentration of a pollutant may be poor, if this pollutant has low fluorescence efficiency in comparison with that typical of a given "generalized" class. Nevertheless, in this case concentration of "generalized" pollutant may also be estimated.

7.4. Results

13 SFS of different pollutants and 6 SFS of different DOMs were used for preparation of patterns during training of a NN "generalized" classifier. All possible combinations of "generalized" classes were allowed for mixture preparation. Thus the trained NN could recognize correctly mixtures of pollutants from up to four "generalized" classes. After presentation of some pattern the system should determine concentrations of detected " generalized" pollutants in the mixture. To solve this task, a set of 15 linear NNs was trained. Each linear NN corresponds to one of the 15 possible combinations of 4 "generalized" classes detected in the presented mixture: 4 NNs for each class, 6 NNs for all pairs of classes ("double mixtures"), 4 NNs for all triads of classes ("triple mixtures"), and 1 NN for simultaneous activity of all classes ("quadruple mixtures").

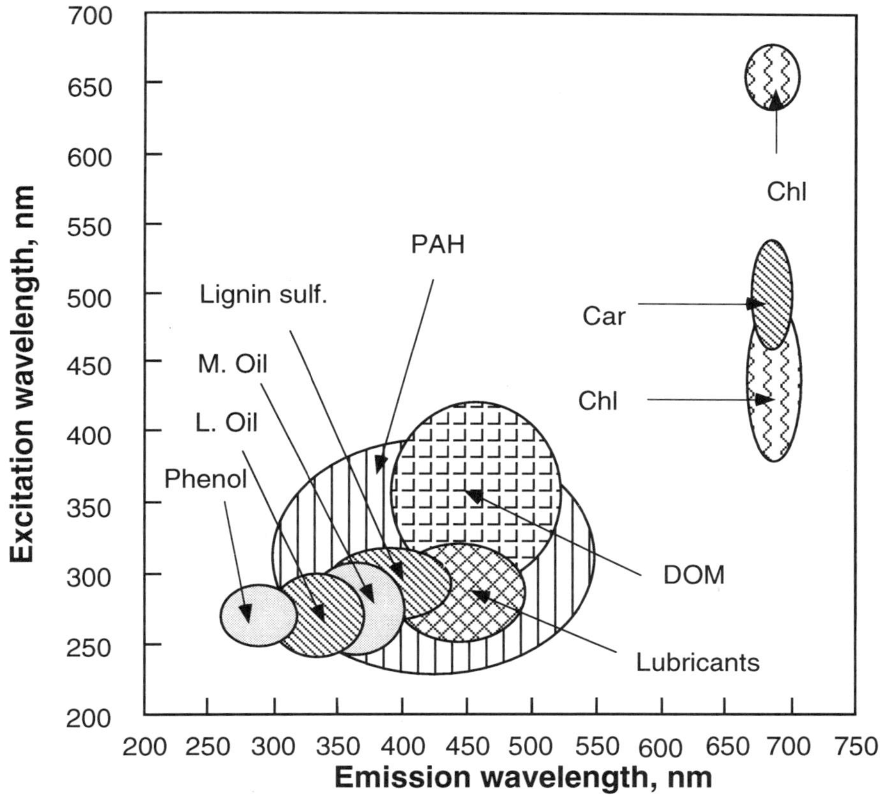

Figure 7.4. Regions of maximum fluorescence for different technogeneous pollutants and natural substances (L. Oil - light oil products, M. Oil - medium oil products, Lignin sulf. - lignin sulphanates, PAH - polyaromatic hydrocarbonates, DOM - dissolved organic matter, Chl - chlorophyll, Car - carotinoids).

Typical minimal detectable pollutant concentrations and accuracy of concentrations determination for the system working with "generalized" classes are presented in the Table 7.1. Two values of DOM concentration correspond approximately to the low and high limits of possible DOM concentrations. Accuracy of concentration determination for different types of mixtures of "generalized" classes is presented in the Table 7.2.

For comparison, in the Table 7.3 minimal detectable pollutant concentrations typical for the system configured to work on the basis of end-user library (i.e. with identification of pollutant) are presented.[6]

One can see that accuracy and sensitivity of the system using "generalized" classes are not as good as the ones typical of the system with pollutant identification.

Nevertheless, the possibility of recognizing complex mixtures of pollutants, and wide range of pollutants that can be classified under such approach, make this system very attractive.

Table 7.1: Minimal detectable concentration and accuracy of concentration determination for "generalized" classes.

"Generalized" class of pollutant	Minimal detectable concentration of pollutant, ppm, for DOM conc., mg/l organic carbon		Accuracy of concentration determination, ppm
	0.3	10	
Phenols	0.06 - 0.15	3 - 5	0.2
Light oil products	0.2 - 0.4	6 - 14	0.3
Medium oil products	0.1 - 0.4	4 - 13	0.25
Lubricants	0.05 - 0.25	3 - 10	0.3

Table 7.2: Accuracy of concentration determination for different types of mixtures of "generalized" classes.

Type of mixture of pollutants	Accuracy of concentration determination, ppm
Double	0.4 - 1.0
Triple	0.43 - 1.4
Quadruple	1.7

Table 7.3: Minimal detectable concentration for different types of pollutants (system with identification of pollutant).[6] Concentrations of pollutants are determined with a typical accuracy of 0.05 ppm.

Type of pollutant	Minimal detectable concentration of pollutant, ppm, for DOM conc., mg/l organic carbon	
	0.3	**10**
Phenols	< 0.1	0.5 - 0.8
Light oil products	0.5 - 0.75	1 - 3
Medium oil products	0.13 - 0.5	0.5 - 5
Lubricants	0.1 - 1	0.75 - 10

7.5. Conclusions

The suggested system is able to detect and to classify organic pollution in natural and technogeneous environment. The performance of the system is made insensitive to the DOM spectrum variations. The system gives an adequate answer to presentation of SFS corresponding to mixtures of pollutants. For "generalized" classes, the system is able to classify up to quadruple mixture of pollutants from different classes, and concentrations of the pollutants in the mixture are determined by a linear NN that is selected according to the detected combination of classes.

Future development of the system comprises automatic determination of optimal separation of pollutants into classes used by hierarchical structure, and automatic adjustment of an existing structure to end-user library expansion.

7.6. References

1. A.E. Dudelzak, S.M. Babichenko, L.V. Poryvkina and K.U. Saar, "Total luminescent spectroscopy for remote laser diagnostics of natural water conditions," *Appl. Opt.* **30** (1991) 453-458.
2. L.V. Poryvkina, S.M. Babichenko J.J. and Lapimaa, "Spectral variability of humus substance in marine ecosystems," *AMBIO* **21** (1992) 465-467.
3. R.P. Lippman, "An Introduction to Computing with Neural Nets," *IEEE ASSP Mag.* (1987) 4-22.
4. D.E. Rumelhart, G.E. Hinton and R.J. Williams, *Parallel Distributed Processing, Explorations in the Microstructures of Cognition, 1: Foundations* (MIT Press, Cambridge, MA, 1986), pp. 318-362.
5. Y.V. Orlov, I.G. Persiantsev and S.P. Rebrik, "Application of neural networks to fluorescent diagnostics of organic pollution in natural waters," *RNNS/IEEE Symposium on Neuroinformatics and Neurocomputers*, (Rostov-on-Don, 1992), pp. 763-773.
6. Y.V. Orlov, I.G. Persiantsev, S.P. Rebrik, "Application of neural networks to fluorescent diagnostics of organic pollution in natural waters," *Proc.1993 IEEE Int. Conf. on Neural Networks* (San Francisco, California, March 28-April 1, 1993), pp. 1230-1235.

8. RELIABILITY AND RISK ANALYSIS USING ARTIFICIAL NEURAL NETWORKS

DAVID G. ROBINSON
Manufacturing Systems Reliability Department, Sandia National Laboratories†*, PO Box 5800*
Albuquerque, New Mexico 87185-0746, USA
E-mail: drobin@sandia.gov

ABSTRACT

This paper discusses preliminary research at Sandia National Laboratories into the application of artificial neural networks for reliability and risk analysis. The goal of this effort is to develop a reliability based methodology that captures the complex relationship between uncertainty in material properties and manufacturing processes and the resulting uncertainty in life prediction estimates. The inputs to the neural network model are probability density functions describing system characteristics and the output is a statistical description of system performance. The most recent application of this methodology involves the comparison of various low-residue, lead-free soldering processes with the desire to minimize the associated waste streams with no reduction in product reliability. Model inputs include statistical descriptions of various material properties such as the coefficients of thermal expansion of solder and substrate. Consideration is also given to stochastic variation in the operational environment to which the electronic components might be exposed. Model output includes a probabilistic characterization of the fatigue life of the surface mounted component.

8.1. Introduction

This paper discusses an alternative to the parametrically based methods for modeling the fatigue life of a solder connection. One of the more popular parametric expressions for fatigue life is the Coffin-Manson relationship. However, this function relates various parameters to the *median* fatigue life and therefore is limited in applications where reliability of solder joints is a concern. This is a concern since it is possible for two alloys to have different life characteristics and yet have the same median fatigue life.

Clearly, it is difficult to capture the complex nature of the fatigue process with such simple parametric expressions. Alternatively, an advantage of neural networks over classical modeling methods is the increased accuracy in characterizing complex failure processes. However, a major benefit of using parametric methods is the ability to model the uncertainty in the failure process and identification of those design parameters that significantly impact the reliability of the solder joint. This has typi-

---

†This work was supported by the U.S. Department of Energy under Contract DE-AC04-94AL85000.

cally been explored using first or second order reliability methods in conjunction with a parametric based model such as the Coffin-Manson.

A major draw back in using first or second order reliability methods is that they assume that the parametric relationship characterizes the process being considered with absolute accuracy. However, estimation of this function is typically approximate at best and often, as in the case of the Coffin-Manson relationship, requires the introduction of 'fudge' factors to improve the accuracy of the model.

While neural networks are generally more accurate in modeling complex input/output relationships, neural networks have been limited to deterministic input (or a series of random realizations) and deterministic output. This has limited their usefulness in the identification of those input parameters that are significantly contributing to uncertainty in the output. In modeling the life-length characteristics of solder connections, neural networks can be expected to provide an optimum estimate of the *median* fatigue life, but have been of little use in characterizing the reliability.

The suggested alternative involves a combination of experimental design, neural nets and probabilistic design theory. The initial design space is established using experimental design principles. With this set of input parameters (or training set), a neural network is developed as an accurate model of the manufacturing process. Finally, probabilistic design theory is applied to this model and is used to identify those manufacturing process parameters that are contributing to variability in the manufacturing output.

The advantage of the proposed method over classical methods is that a more accurate model representation results and there is therefore increased accuracy in predicting the expected life characteristics of the failure process. Fundamentally, the approach provides a direct link between the experimental results and the reliability analysis; the reliability analysis is not restricted by the assumption of a particular functional form of the expected fatigue life. The experimental data drives life prediction rather than some arbitrary parametric function.

8.2. Neural Networks Background

Definition of Terms:

$w_{i,j,k}$	weight between node j in layer $(k-1)$ and node i in layer k
$I_{i,k}$	input to node i in layer k
$O_{i,k}$	output of node i in layer k
z_i	$I_{i,1}$, input to the network at node i
y_i	$O_{i,n}$, observed output of the network at node i
$\theta_{i,k}$	parameter chosen to control the maximum output from node i (>0)

$\beta_{i,k}$ parameter chosen to control the slope of the input/output sigmoid (>0)

n_i number of nodes in layer I

Artificial neural networks are an attempt to mimic the processes used by the human mind to construct models of very complex systems. Such networks have been successfully applied since the early 1970's to a variety of problems. Of particular interest is the recent suggestion that they can be used as alternatives to statistical methods for modeling a number of manufacturing process.[1-3]

A typical neural network consists of k layers of nodes. Each layer consists of n_k nodes each of which is connected to each of the nodes in the layers immediately above and below. Information in the form of an input vector $\mathbf{z}$ is processed forward to each successive layer until the final output is available. The network output is compared to the desired output and the resulting error is processed backward through the network and the model is adjusted. This *training* cycle continues until the error achieves some minimum criteria. This type of neural network model is commonly referred to as a feed-forward error back-propagation model and is one of the most common structures used in the design of a network.

For a three layer, backpropagation system, with only one output, the following partial differential equations can be developed:

$$\begin{aligned}\frac{\partial y}{\partial z_j} &= O_{j,1}\left(\frac{O_{j,1}}{\theta_{j,1}}-1\right)\beta_{j,1}\sum_{r=1}^{n_2}\gamma_{1,r,2}w_{r,j,2}\\ \gamma_{1,r,2} &= O_{r,2}\left(\frac{O_{r,2}}{\theta_{r,2}}-1\right)\beta_{r,2}\sum_{s=1}^{n_3=1}\gamma_{1,s,3}w_{s,r,3}\\ &= O_{r,2}\left(\frac{O_{r,2}}{\theta_{r,2}}-1\right)\beta_{r,2}\gamma_{1,1,3}w_{1,r,3}\end{aligned} \tag{8.1}$$

and:

$$\gamma_{1,1,3} = y\left(\frac{y}{\theta_{1,3}}-1\right)\beta_{1,3} \tag{8.2}$$

These partial derivatives will be an integral element in the probabilistic design phase of the analysis.

8.3. Probabilistic Design Background

Given a failure process with parameters: $\mathbf{z}=(z_1, z_2,\ldots, z_m)$. The fatigue process is observed and the response, e.g. cycles to failure, is measured and recorded. The objective is to identify, and subsequently influence, those parameters which are significantly contributing to the variability in the life-length characteristics. Through the identification of these factors and their subsequent control, the uncertainty in the system response can be decreased and the overall reliability of the soldering process is improved. It will be assumed that the input to the neural network, $\mathbf{z}$, is a realization from an m dimensional random process.

Let $G(\mathbf{z})=0$ be a function describing the performance of the system. This function partitions the design space into a region where combinations of $\mathbf{z}$ result in acceptable system performance, $G(\mathbf{z})>0$, and combinations where system performance is unacceptable, $G(\mathbf{z})<0$. The hyper surface defined by $G(\mathbf{z})=0$ is generally referred to as the *limit state surface*. For the two dimensional case it is clear that, if z_1 and z_2 are random variables with joint probability density function $f(z_1, z_2)$, even though the mean behavior of the system is clearly acceptable, there is a finite probability that there will be realization of these two variables that will result in unacceptable performance. An exact evaluation of the probability of this event is available through the solution of the m-dimensional integral:

$$\Pr\{\text{unacceptable performance}\} = p_u = \iint \ldots \int f(z_1, z_2, \ldots, z_m) dz_1 dz_2 \ldots dz_m \quad (8.3)$$

Solution of this integral can be a very difficult task except in the very simplest of situations. An alternative is an approximate solution available through the use of first order probabilistic design methods. Given the distance from the origin to the failure surface: $d = \left(\mathbf{z}^{\mathrm{T}}\mathbf{z}\right)^{1/2}$ define the index β:

$$\beta = \min_{z} d = \left(\mathbf{z}^{\mathrm{T}}\mathbf{z}\right)^{1/2} \quad (8.4)$$

$$\text{subject to: } G(\mathbf{z}) = 0$$

The point $\mathbf{z}^* = \left(z_1^*, z_2^*, \ldots, z_m^*\right)$ on the failure surface which is identified as closest to the origin is referred to as the most probable point. An approximate expression for the risk of being in the unacceptable region can then be shown to be: $risk = \Phi(-\beta)$, where $\Phi(-\beta)$ is the standardized Gaussian density function evaluated at $-\beta$.

Define the gradient vector:

$$\nabla = \left(\frac{\partial G}{\partial z_1}, \frac{\partial G}{\partial z_2}, \ldots, \frac{\partial G}{\partial z_m}\right) \quad (8.5)$$

It can be shown that the minimum distance from the origin to the limit state surface is given by the expression:[4]

$$\beta = \frac{-\nabla^{*}\mathbf{z}^{*}}{(\nabla^{*T}\nabla^{*})^{1/2}}$$

$$= \frac{-\sum z_i^{*}\left(\frac{\partial G}{\partial z_i}\right)_{z=z^{*}}}{\left[\sum\left(\frac{\partial G}{\partial z_i}\right)^2_{z=z^{*}}\right]^{1/2}} \tag{8.6}$$

Where the mean and standard deviation of $G(\mathbf{z})$ are approximately:

$$\mu \cong -\nabla^{*}\mathbf{z}^{*}$$
$$\sigma \cong (\nabla^{*T}\nabla^{*})^{1/2} \tag{8.7}$$

To find the point $\mathbf{z}^{*} = (z_1^{*}, z_2^{*}, \ldots, z_m^{*})$ an iterative procedure can be incorporated. It should be noted that a subtle, but significant difference from traditional methods is that $\mathbf{z}^{*} \neq (\mu_{z_1}, \mu_{z_2}, \ldots, \mu_{z_n})$. A number of schemes can be employed to find those values of $\mathbf{z}^{*}$ that minimizes the distance to the limit state surface and thus the index β. For well behaved $G(\mathbf{z})$ where multiple solutions are unlikely, a simple calculus based search algorithm, such as a that described above, can be used. Alternatively, if the limit state function is particularly complicated, the use of genetic algorithms has been successfully applied.[6]

8.4. Relationship to Neural Networks

From our previous discussion, it is clear that the neural network represents the function $G(\mathbf{z}) = y(\mathbf{z})$ and the gradient vector above can be expressed:

$$\nabla_{z^{*}} = \left(\frac{\partial y}{\partial z_1^{*}}, \frac{\partial y}{\partial z_2^{*}}, \ldots, \frac{\partial y}{\partial z_m^{*}}\right) \tag{8.8}$$

and the index β is therefore:

$$\beta = \frac{-\nabla^{T}_{\mathbf{z}^{*}}\mathbf{z}^{*}}{(\nabla^{T}_{\mathbf{z}^{*}}\nabla_{\mathbf{z}^{*}})^{1/2}} \tag{8.9}$$

Following the solution of the index β, the most probable point can then be decomposed: $z_i^{*} = -\alpha_i\beta$. Where the direction cosines:

$$\alpha = \frac{-\nabla^{T}_{\mathbf{z}^{*}}}{(\nabla^{T}_{\mathbf{z}^{*}}\nabla_{\mathbf{z}^{*}})^{1/2}} \tag{8.10}$$

indicate the relative contribution of the *i*th variable to the probability of failure p_u and are often referred to as the importance factors. Those process parameters associated with large importance factors will be those parameters significantly contributing to uncertainty in the fatigue process. It should be noted these importance factors are generally not available when traditional Monte Carlo based methods are applied.

8.5. Application

The specific application of the above methodology involves the characterization of the fatigue life of a solder joint. Of particular interest will be the reliability of new environmentally friendly solder alloys being developed. While a number of solder joint failure mechanisms are possible, the dominate mode for surface mount solder joint reliability is fatigue damage resulting from cyclic differential thermal expansion. This damage mechanism results primarily from thermal expansion differences between the component, solder and substrate materials. These differences induce cyclic shear strains which in turn lead to an accumulation of fatigue damage. A relationship commonly used to describe the *expected* fatigue life of a solder joint in this environment is the Coffin-Manson relationship:

$$N_f = \frac{1}{2}\left(\frac{\Delta\gamma}{2\varepsilon_f}\right)^{1/c} \tag{8.11}$$

Define the following parameters:

N_f $\equiv$ Mean fatigue life

c $\equiv$ fatigue ductility exponent

$= -0.442 - 6\times10^{-4} T_{SJ} + 1.74\times10^{-2}\ln\left(1+\frac{360}{t_D}\right) \approx -.442$

ε_f $\equiv$ fatigue ductility coefficient ≈ 0.325 for eutectic Sn-Pb solder

Δ_γ $\equiv$ cyclic total plastic shear strain range

$= F\frac{L_D}{h}\Delta(\alpha\Delta T)$

F $\equiv$ fudge factor to account for inaccuracies in model ≈ 1.0

$2L_D$ $\equiv$ maximum distance between solder joints = 1200 *mils*

h $\equiv$ solder joint height = 8 *mils*

$\Delta(\alpha\Delta T)$ $\equiv$ absolute cyclic differential thermal expansion between component / substrate solder

$= \Delta\alpha\Delta T$

$\Delta\alpha$ $= |\alpha_s - \alpha_{CS}|$

α_s, α_{CS} ≡ coefficients of thermal expansion (CTE) for solder and component / substrate

ΔT ≡ cyclic temperature swing

The major source of fatigue damage results from the CTE differences between the solder and the component and substrate. The following discussion outlines the fundamentals of the validation of the modeling and analysis approach used.

Since experimental data are not available at this time, an artificial data set was simulated under the assumption that the Coffin-Manson relationship in some sense characterizes the fatigue process. Preliminary investigations have been of limited scope to permit a tractable validation. Specifically, the fatigue life will be assumed to follow a simplified Coffin-Manson relationship where only α_S, α_{CS} and ΔT are considered sources of uncertainty.

These parameters are assumed to be lognormally distributed random variables with the following statistical properties:

$$\begin{aligned} \alpha_s &\sim Ln(\tilde{\alpha}_s = 6\times10^{-6}\ \text{ppm}/\text{C}^\circ, C_s = 0.2) \\ \alpha_{CS} &\sim Ln(\tilde{\alpha}_C = 25\times10^{-6}\,\text{ppm}/\text{C}^\circ, C_C = 0.2) \\ \Delta T &\sim Ln(\tilde{T}_T = 100\ \text{C}^\circ, C_T = 0.5) \end{aligned} \tag{8.12}$$

where $\tilde{\alpha}_s, \tilde{\alpha}_C$, and $\Delta\tilde{T}$ are the median values of the parameters and C_s, C_C,and C_T are the associated coefficients of variation. Given these modeling assumptions we can simulate test data for training and exercising the neural network model.

A total of twenty seven random values each of the three CTE's and cyclic temperature ranges were generated. Twenty seven was chosen since the actual data would presumably result from exercising a full factorial experimental design of three factors each at three levels. Each of these combinations was input to the Coffin-Manson relationship and an 'observed' fatigue life calculated. The data is then used to train a feed-forward error back-propagation neural network.

8.6. Neural Network Model

The NN model of the fatigue process is depicted in Figure 8.1. The topology is rather straightforward with only three layers: three input nodes, one hidden layer and one output node. Each of the input nodes corresponds to α_S, α_{CS} and ΔT respectively, while the output corresponds to the estimated fatigue life. Using the 27 input vectors, the model is trained to an acceptable level and the connection weights estimated. The result of this step is a neural network model of the relationship between the solder joint design and operational parameters and the fatigue life of the joint.

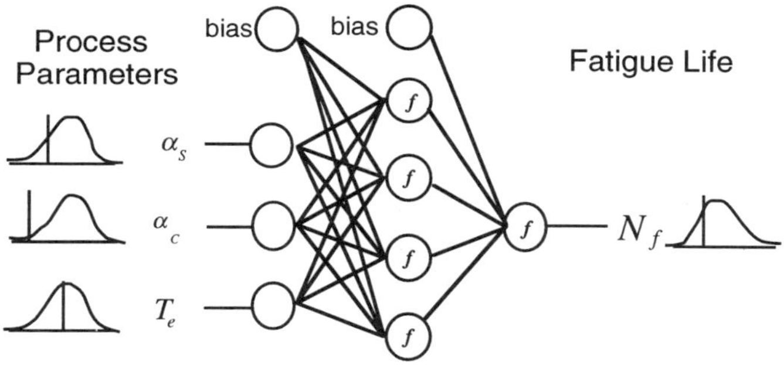

Figure 8.1. Example of Neural Network of Fatigue Process

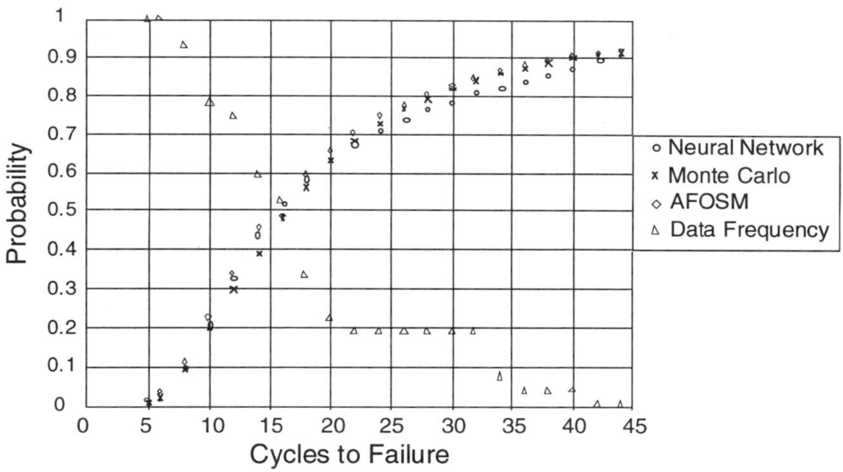

Figure 8.2. Probability of Solder Connection Failure

8.7. Results

Once the interconnection weights have been established from the training process, the ANN accurately transforms combinations of input vectors to the expected output. The network topology, when combined with these weights, provides all the information necessary to estimate the required partial derivatives, the most probable point, an estimate of the safety index and finally the probability of failure. Figure 8.2 summarize the results of one such investigation. This figure contrasts the results from an advanced first-order, second-moment risk analysis, the results from the new ANN approach and finally the results from a Monte Carlo simulation.

Also presented in Figure 8.2 is the density of the sample input data. Note that over 80% of the simulated times-to-failure occur between 0 and 22 cycles to failure. Out of the 27 data simulated data sets, only 5 resulted in failures greater than 22 cycles. Since there was very limited data upon which to train the ANN, this is an area where the greatest error between the Monte Carlo results and the ANN occurs. However, the AFOSM method depends only on the assumption of a particular function and, once this function is estimated, is independent of the amount of data available. In defense of the ANN method, the analyst also runs the risk of choosing a poor underlying functional relationship.

8.8. Conclusions

The goal of this effort was to develop an alternative reliability analysis methodology that:

- Permits material characteristics of the solder alloys and substrate, as well as geometry of the solder connection, to be included in the analysis. Characteristics included are currently limited to coefficients of thermal expansion of substrate and alloy
- Does not require a presupposed form for the relationship between the model parameters and the response of the system. Typically, a specific functional form is assumed based primarily on historical literature rather than strong physical or empirical evidence.
- Captures relationship between uncertainty in material properties and manufacturing processes and uncertainty in fatigue life estimates.

Characterizing the reliability of a solder connection has historically been based upon some variation of the Coffin-Manson relationship. This function relates a variety of dimensional, material and environmental characteristics to the expected fatigue life of the connections. However, it has been increasingly evident in the literature that various 'fudge factors' must be applied to get a good match between this relationship and actual test data.

In addition to potential inaccuracies associated with assuming a particular functional form, the approach provides at best an estimate of the expected life of a solder connection. The mean alone provides almost no useful information with which to compare various solder alloys. One reason for this is that the Coffin-Manson approach is extremely limited in dealing with information about the material properties of the solder alloys beyond coefficients of thermal expansion. Preliminary results indicate that neural networks hold the promise of more accurately characterizing the complex process and can be extended to include uncertainty in the process parameters.

8.9. References

1. S. Rangwala and D. Dornfeld, "Learning and Optimization of Machining Operations Using Computing Abilities of Neural Networks," *IEEE Trans Systems, Man, and Cybernetics* **19** (1989) 299-314.
2. C. Himmel and G. May, "Advantages of Plasma Etch Modeling Using Neural Networks Over Statistical Techniques," *IEEE Trans Semiconductor Manuf.* **6** (1993) 103-111.
3. F. Nadi, A. Agonio and D. Hodges, "Use of Influence Diagrams and Neural Networks in Modeling Semiconductor Manufacturing Processes," *IEEE Trans Semiconductor Manuf.* **4** (1991) 52-58.
4. M. Shinozuka, "Basic Analysis of Structural Safety," *J. of Structural Division ASCE* **3** (March 1983) 109.
5. D. Robinson and G. Toussaint, "Reliability of Unidirectional Composites Using Genetic Algorithms," in *Probabilistic Structural Mechanics: Advances in Structural Reliability Methods*, ed.s P. Spanos, Y.-T. Wu (Springer-Verlag, 1994).

9. ELECTRONIC NOSES AND THEIR APPLICATIONS IN ENVIRONMENTAL MONITORING

SHERIF HASHEM, PAUL E. KELLER, LARS J. KANGAS
Pacific Northwest National Laboratory†*, P.O. Box 999, MS K1-87*
Richland, Washington 99352, USA
E-mail: s_hashem@pnl.gov, pe_keller@pnl.gov, lj_kangas@pnl.gov

and

RICHARD T. KOUZES
Department of Physics, West Virginia University, P.O. Box 6216, 302 Stewart Hall
Morgantown, West Virginia 26505, USA
E-mail: rkouzes@wvnvm.wvnet.edu

ABSTRACT

Compact, portable systems capable of quickly identifying contaminants in the field are of great importance when monitoring the environment. In this paper, we examine the effectiveness of using artificial neural networks for real-time data analysis of a sensor array. Analyzing the sensor data in parallel may allow for rapid identification of contaminants in the field without requiring highly selective component sensors. A sensor array combined with a data analysis module is referred to as an *electronic nose*.

In this paper, we investigate the trade off between sensor sensitivity and selectivity relating to the applications of neural network based-electronic noses in environmental monitoring. We use a prototype electronic nose which consists of nine tin-oxide Taguchi-type sensors, a temperature sensor, and a humidity sensor. We illustrate that by using neural network based analysis of a sensor data, the selectivity of a sensor array may be significantly improved, especially when some (or all) sensors are not highly selective.

Keywords: neural network, sensor array, environmental monitoring, sensor selectivity.

9.1 Introduction

One of the missions of the Pacific Northwest National Laboratory is to examine and develop new technologies for environmental restoration and waste management

---

†This work was supported by the Associated Western Universities, Inc., Northwest Division under Grant DE-FG06-89ER-75522 with the U.S. Department of Energy, by the Environmental Molecular Sciences Laboratory construction project, and by the Laboratory Directed Research and Development program at Pacific Northwest National Laboratory (PNNL). PNNL is a multiprogram national laboratory operated by Battelle Memorial Institute for the U.S. Department of Energy under Contract DE-AC06-76RLO 1830.

at the U.S. Department of Energy's Hanford Site[1] (a former plutonium production facility). Enormous amounts of hazardous waste were generated during more than 40 years of plutonium production at the Hanford Site. There is an estimated 1700 waste sites distributed around the 1450 square kilometers (560 square miles) of southeastern Washington state (USA) that comprise the Hanford Site. This waste includes nuclear waste (e.g., fission products), toxic chemical waste (e.g., carbon tetrachloride, ferrocyanide, nitrates, etc.), and mixed waste (combined radioactive and chemical waste). The current mission at the Hanford Site is environmental restoration and waste management.

As part of this mission, the Pacific Northwest National Laboratory is exploring the technologies required to perform environmental restoration and waste management in a cost effective manner. This effort includes the development of portable, inexpensive systems capable of real-time identification of contaminants in the field. The objective of our research is to demonstrate the potential information processing capabilities of the neural network paradigm in sensor analysis.

A difficult problem in identifying contaminants in the field is the need for highly sensitive and selective sensors, which are often expensive and sometimes difficult to achieve.[2] This led to research on sensor arrays compromising a set of sensors whose responses are collectively analyzed.[2-4] When a sensor array is analyzed in parallel, more analytes can be identified than by relying separately on the individual sensors.[3]

The use of artificial neural networks (ANNs) for analyzing sensor data allows for real-time parallel processing of the data. Artificial neural networks are widely used in data processing applications where real-time data analysis and information extraction are required. One advantage of the neural network approach is that most of the intense computation takes place during the training process. Once the ANN is trained for a particular task, operation is relatively fast. Real-time classification of unknown samples mainly involves simple matrix manipulation and application of look-up tables (activation function). Thus, unknown samples can be rapidly identified in the field.

9.2. Sensor Data Analysis

There are many real-time (rapid response) and remote sensing applications that require an inexpensive, compact, and automated system for identifying an object (e.g., target, chemical, isotope). Such a system can be built by combining a sensor array with an ANN. A generic system is shown in Figure 9.1.

The quantity and complexity of the data collected by sensor arrays can make conventional analysis of data difficult. ANNs, which have been used to analyze complex data and for pattern recognition, could be a better choice for sensor data analysis. A common approach in sensor analysis is to build an array of sensors, where each sensor in the array is designed to respond to a specific analyte. With this approach, the number of sensors must be at least as great as the number of analytes being monitored. When an ANN is combined with a sensor array, the number of detectable analytes is generally greater than the number of sensors.[3] A sensor array is composed of several sensing elements, where each element measures a different property of the sensed sample. Each object (e.g., target, chemical, isotope) presented to the sensor array produces a signature or pattern characteristic of the object. By presenting many different objects to the sensor array, a database of signatures can be built up. From this database, training sets and test sets are generated. These sets are collections of labeled patterns (signatures) representative of the desired identification mapping. The training sets are used to configure the ANNs. The goal of this training is to learn an association between the sensor array patterns and the labels representing the data.

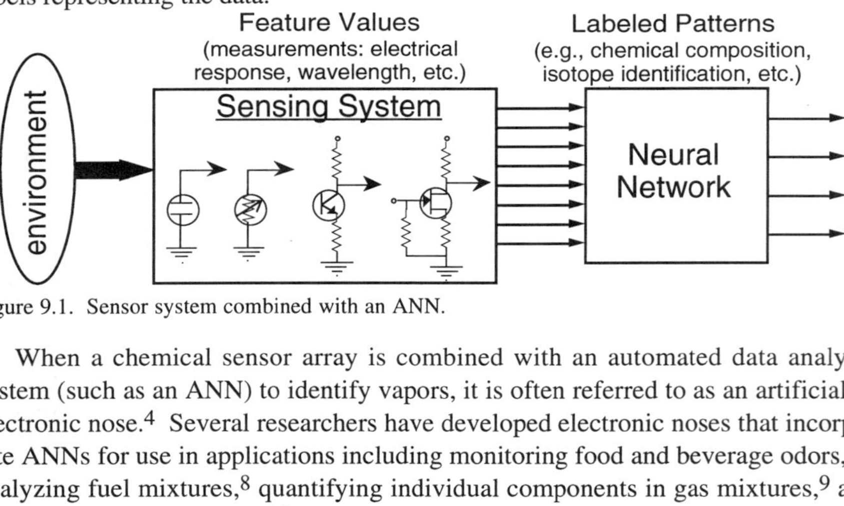

Figure 9.1. Sensor system combined with an ANN.

When a chemical sensor array is combined with an automated data analysis system (such as an ANN) to identify vapors, it is often referred to as an artificial or electronic nose.[4] Several researchers have developed electronic noses that incorporate ANNs for use in applications including monitoring food and beverage odors,[5-7] analyzing fuel mixtures,[8] quantifying individual components in gas mixtures,[9] and environmental monitoring.[10] Several ANN configurations have been used in electronic noses including backpropagation-trained, feed-forward networks; Kohonen's self-organizing networks; Boltzmann machines; and Hopfield networks.[11] This paper extends the work by Keller[10] *et al.* in the area of environmental monitoring. We here examine some aspects relating to identifying mixtures of analytes.

9.3. A Prototype Chemical Vapor Sensing System

This system consists of an array of nine tin-oxide gas sensors, a humidity sensor, and a temperature sensor to examine the environment. Although each sensor is designed for a specific chemical, each responds to a wide variety of chemical vapors. Collectively, these sensors respond with unique signatures (patterns) to different chemicals. During the training process, various chemicals with known mixtures are presented to the system. In the initial studies, the backpropagation algorithm was used to train the ANN to provide the correct analysis of the presented chemicals.

The nine tin-oxide sensors are commercially available Taguchi-type gas sensors obtained from Figaro Co. Ltd. (Sensor 1, TGS 109; Sensors 2 and 3, TGS 822; Sensor 4, TGS 813; Sensor 5, TGS 821; Sensor 6, TGS 824; Sensor 7, TGS 825; Sensor 8, TGS 842; and Sensor 9, TGS 880). Exposure of a tin-oxide sensor to a vapor produces a large change in its electrical resistance.[12] The humidity sensor (Sensor 10: NH-02) and the temperature sensor (Sensor 11: 5KD-5) are used to monitor the conditions of the experiment and are also fed into the ANN.

An ANN was constructed as a multilayer feedforward network and was trained with the backpropagation of error algorithm[13] by using a training set from the sensor database. The network has one hidden layer with four hidden units. The activation function for the hidden units as well as the output units is the logistic sigmoid function $g(s) = (1 + e^{-s})^{-1}$. The training set consists of 177 patterns which corresponds to five household chemicals: acetone, ammonia, isopropanol alcohol, lighter fluid, and vinegar. We used another category, "none," to denote the absence of all chemicals except those normally found in the air. This resulted in six output categories from the ANN. Figure 9.2 illustrates the network layout.

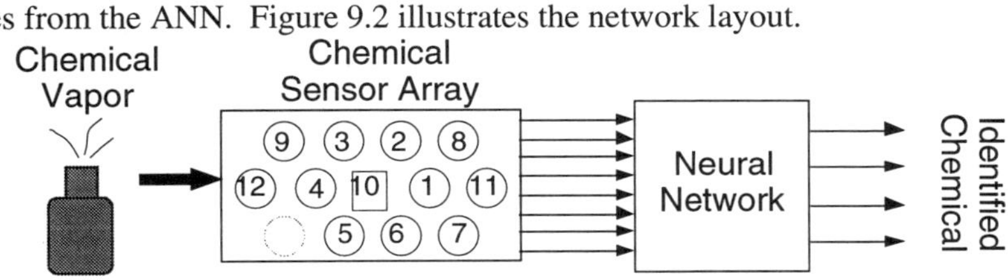

Figure 9.2. ANN used to identify household chemicals.

During operation, the sensor array "smells" a vapor, the sensor signals are digitized and fed into a computer, and the ANN (implemented in software) then identifies the chemical. This identification time is limited only by the response time of the chemical sensors, which is on the order of a few seconds.

9.4. Discussion and Conclusions

Figures 9.4 and 9.5 illustrate the responses of the sensors and the ANN classification for a variety of test chemicals presented to the network (shown in Figure 9.3). The network was able to correctly classify the test samples, with small residual errors.

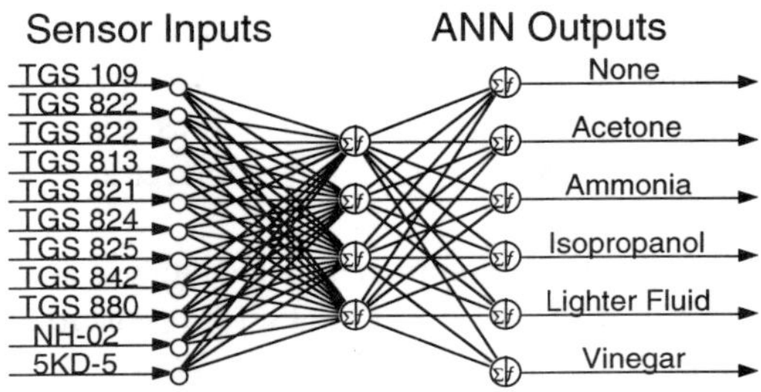

Figure 9.3. Network Structure.

While the ANN used here was not trained to quantify the concentration level of the identified analytes, it was trained with samples which have different concentrations of the analytes. This allowed the network to generalize well on the test data set.

From the responses of the sensors to the analytes, one can easily see that the individual sensors in the array are not selective (Figure 9.4). In addition, when a mixture of two or more chemicals is presented to the sensor array, the resultant pattern (sensor values) may be even harder to analyze (see Figure 9.5: c, d, and e). Thus, analyzing the sensor responses separately may not be adequate to yield the classification accuracy achieved by analyzing the data in parallel.

These results demonstrate the pattern recognition capabilities of the neural network paradigm in sensor analysis, especially when the individual sensors are not highly selective. Besides, the prototype presented here has several advantages for real-world applications including compactness, portability, real-time analysis, and automation. Further work will involve comparing neural network sensor analysis to more conventional techniques, exploring other neural network paradigms, and evolving the preliminary prototypes to field systems.

Information on ANN developments at Pacific Northwest National Laboratory is available in the World Wide Web (WWW) pages of the Environmental Molecular Sciences Laboratory.

URL: http://www.emsl.pnl.gov:2080/docs/cie/neural/

9.5. References

1. B G. Levi, "Hanford Seeks Short- and Long-term Solutions to its Legacy of Waste," *Physics Today* **45(3)** (March 1992) pp. 17-21.
2. S.J. Patrash and E.T. Zellers, "Characterization of Polymeric Surface Acoustic Wave Sensor Coatings and Semiempirical Models of Sensor Responses to Organic Vapors," *Anal. Chem* **65** (1993) 2055-2066.

3. B.S. Hoffheins, "Using Sensor Arrays and Pattern Recognition to Identify Organic Compounds," *MS-Thesis*, (The University of Tennessee, Knoxville, TN, 1989).
4. J.W. Gardner, E.L. Hines and M. Wilkinson., "Application of Artificial Neural Networks to an Electronic Olfactory System," *Measurement Science and Technology* **1** (1990) 446-451.
5. T. Moriizumi, T. Nakamoto and Y. Sakuraba, "Pattern Recognition in Electronic Noses by Artificial Neural Network Models," in *Sensors and Sensory Systems for an Electronic Nose*, ed.s J.W. Gardner and P.N. Bartlett, (Kluweer Academic Publishers, Amsterdam, The Netherlands,, 1992), pp. 217-236.
6. A.M. Pisanelli, A.A. Qutob, P. Travers, S. Szyszko and K.C. Persaud, "Applications of Multiarray Polymer Sensors to Food Industries," *Life Chemistry Reports* **11** (1994) 303-308.
7. S. Nathan, "On the Scent of Something Big," *Chemistry and Industry* (1 August 1994) 587.
8. R.J. Lauf and B.S. Hoffheins, "Analysis of Liquid Fuels Using a Gas Sensor Array," *Fuel* **70** (1991) 935-940.
9. H. Sundgren, F. Winquist, I. Lukkari and I. Lundström, "Artificial Neural Networks and Gas Sensor Arrays: Quantification of Individual Components in a Gas Mixture," *Measurement Science and Technology* **2** (1991) 464-469.
10. P.E. Keller, R.T. Kouzes and L.J. Kangas, "Three Neural Network Based Sensor Systems for Environmental Monitoring," *IEEE Electro94 Conference* (IEEE, Piscataway, NJ, 1994) pp. 378-382.
11. S. Haykin, *Neural Networks: A Comprehensive Foundation*, (IEEE Press, Piscataway, NJ, 1994).
12. Product literature from Figaro USA, Inc., P.O. Box 357, Wilmette, IL 60091, USA.
13. D.E. Rumelhart, G E. Hinton and R.J. Williams, "Learning Internal Representations by Error Propagation," in *Parallel Distributed Processing: Explorations in the Microstructures of Cognition*. Vol. 1, ed.s D.E. Rumelhart and J.L. McClelland (MIT Press, Cambridge, MA, 1986), pp. 318-362.

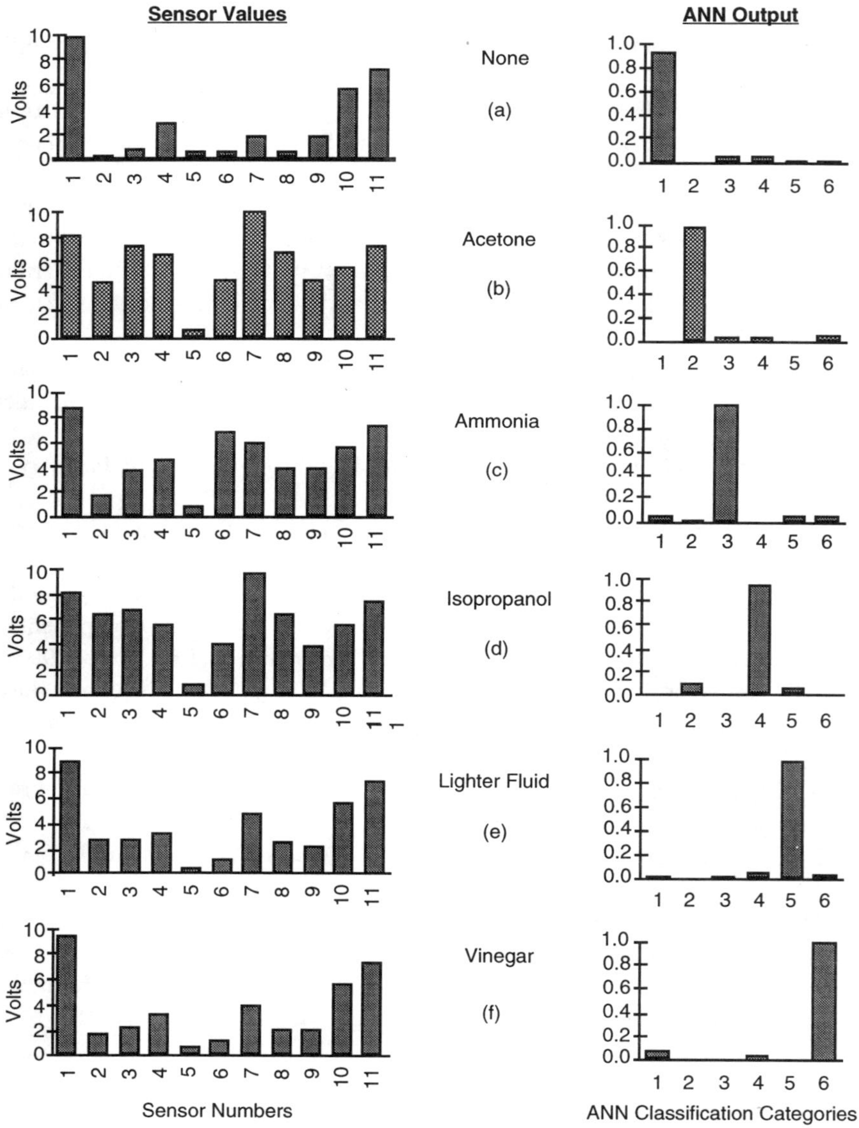

Figure 9.4. Sample responses and ANN classifications I. Sensor numbers and ANN classification categories (on the X-axes) correspond to the ANN in Figure 9.3.

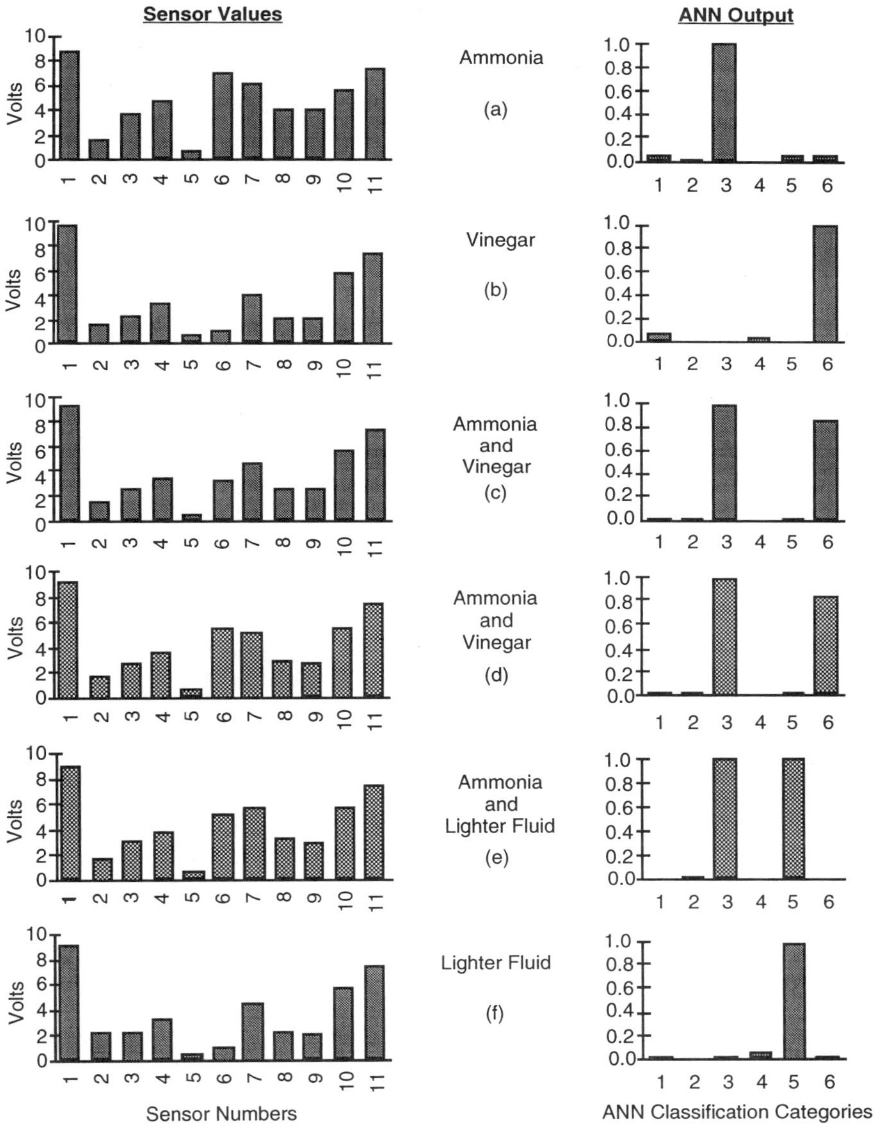

Figure 9.5. Sample responses and ANN classifications II. Sensor numbers and ANN classification categories (on the X-axes) correspond to the ANN in Figure 9.3.

10. APPLICATION OF COMPUTATIONAL NEURAL NETWORKS IN PREDICTING ATMOSPHERIC POLLUTANT CONCENTRATIONS DUE TO FOSSIL-FIRED ELECTRIC POWER GENERATION

FERIAL EL-HAWARY
BH Engineering Systems Limited , P.O. Box 25041
Halifax, Nova Scotia , Canada B3M 4H4
E-mail: elhawary@tuns.ca

and

Technical University of Nova Scotia, P.O. Box 1000
Halifax, Nova Scotia, Canada B3J 2X4

ABSTRACT

This paper deals with the problem of predicting pollution concentration levels at a specific ground location as a result of emissions from fossil electric power generation sources. The level of pollution concentration depends on physical atmospheric conditions (such as wind direction and velocity), stack height, plume rise and selected plume dispersion model. In addition, source pollution concentration levels depend on the active power generation of the units involved.

We report on work in progress employing the Back-propagation model of computational neural networks in order to predict ground level pollution concentration at a specific site. The problem formulation allows the user the choice of using the neural network as either an alarm processor or as a discrete predicting processor. The input pattern consists of site coordinates, plume dispersion model parameters relevant to the site, atmospheric conditions, and active power conditions. Computational experiments with test data demonstrate that the proposed approach is viable.

10.1. Introduction

It is generally acknowledged that computational neural networks (CNN) have been widely applied in many areas of engineering and science. However, not many research results are found on the application of CNN in the area of sensing and predicting pollutants and assessing their environmental impacts. This paper presents an overview of the application to problems of predicting pollution concentration levels at a specific ground location as a result of emissions from fossil electric power generation sources.

A recent search of the literature reveals some related examples. Reference 1, uses a neural network in a rapid system for sea water pollutant diagnosis. Pollutant classification is based on total luminescent spectroscopy (TLS) and is not sensitive to variations in the spectrum of the dissolved organic matter (DOM). The gradual complication of the task during learning is used to reach the minimal decision threshold value. The CNN is successful in presenting a mixture of pollutants spectra, or spectra of unknown substances. Determining pollutant concentration is done in the three steps of classification of a pollutant by the basic net, its identification by an auxiliary net, and concentration determination by a linear neural net with a typical accuracy of 0.05 ppm. It is shown that neural network with two hidden layers for classifying TLS-spectra of low resolution produces classification thresholds close to those of standard TLS-spectra.

The development of an intelligent gas sensor system to identify and quantify hazardous airborne compounds is discussed in Reference 2. Semiconductor gas sensors (SGS) with partially overlapping selectivity have been used as gas detecting devices. Because of its low selectivity, one SGS alone can not accurately specify the type of gas and its actual concentration.

The application of an array of SGS's combined with Kohonen feature map (KFM) neural networks, allows identifying and quantifying unknown species of gases if the gas sensor system has been calibrated earlier using this gas type. The influence of different network parameters, e.g. the number of nodes in the network and the number of pattern vectors used to train the KFM are discussed. The KFM is found to be able to identify all compounds which have been used for calibrating the gas sensor array and for training the KFM.

10.2. The Overall Scheme

The setting for the work presented in this paper is illustrated in Figure 10.1. This is a partial illustration of the ingredients of optimal operation of an electric power system recognizing environmental effects. The first block involves load forecasting for which CNN have been successfully applied.[3] The second block involves the optimal dispatching function whose objectives may be economic or environmental or both. Again, CNN have been successfully applied in this regard. Based on the dispatch results, the power output of each thermal units is adjusted.[4]

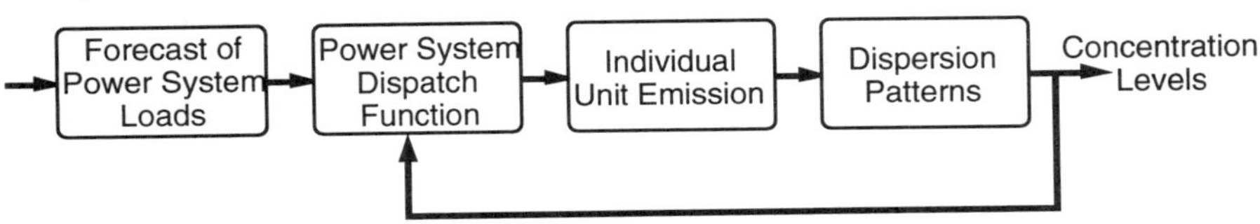

Figure 10.1. Overall Scheme.

The level of emissions such as SO_x and NO_x at the source will of course depend, among other things, on the level of power output of each individual unit. The associated ground concentration of pollutants is determined by the corresponding diffusion process which is dependent on dispersion patterns which in turn depend on meteorological and other conditions. Successful prediction of pollutant concentrations is needed to meet various environmental regulatory requirements. Enhancements to the prediction ability are expected to be achieved by use of CNN. Three opportunities are discussed in this work.

10.3. Principal Plume Dispersion Patterns

The principal patterns of stack gas dispersion are generally classified descriptively in terms of the plume shape and the manner of their dispersion in the ambient atmosphere.[5]

10.3.1. Coning Dispersion Pattern

The effluent plume of the coning model is shaped somewhat like a cone with an extended horizontal axis as shown in Figure 10.2. It generally occurs under near-neutral stability and moderate to high wind speed conditions, on cloudy and windy days or windy nights.

Coning dispersion is identified with maximum surface concentrations for generating plants with ratings up to 200-250 MW, with 75 to 120 m stacks. The level and location of maximum surface concentrations are primarily dependent on the effective stack height (plume rise plus actual stack height), wind speed, and atmospheric stability.

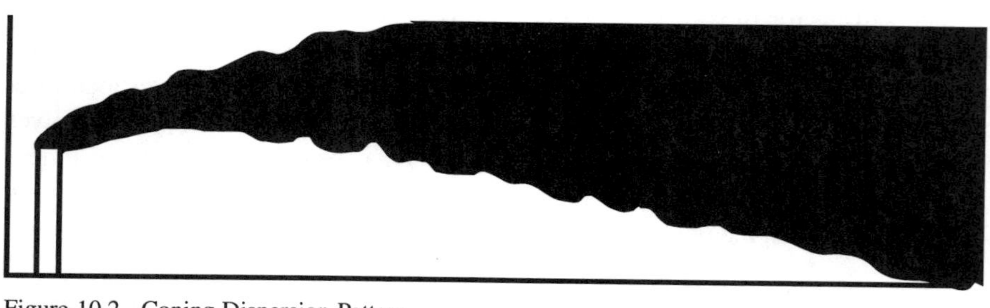

Figure 10.2. Coning Dispersion Pattern.

10.3.2. Fanning and Inversion Breakup

Fanning occurs when a plume is emitted into a stable atmosphere and transported downwind as a compact flat ribbon, i.e. the fanning plume spreading laterally with minimum vertical dispersion.

Inversion breakup occurs when a fanning plume is uniformly dispersed to the ground when thermally induced vertical mixing develops upward through the plume. Maximum surface concentrations from inversion breakup dispersion may be high, but their duration is short, persisting 30-45 min within a relatively narrow band beneath the originally stable plume at distances up to 30 km from source.

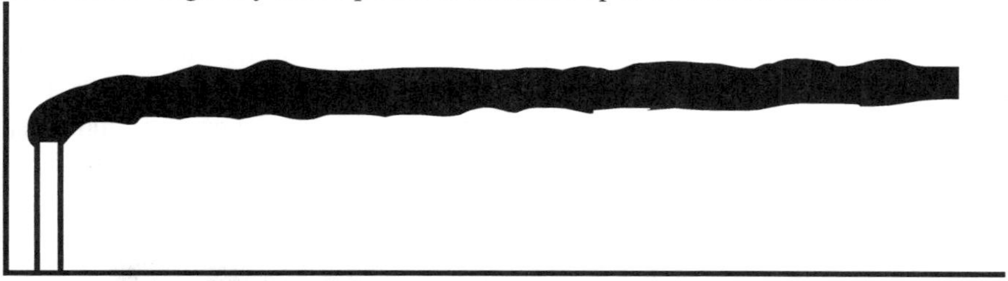

Figure 10.3. Fanning Dispersion Pattern.

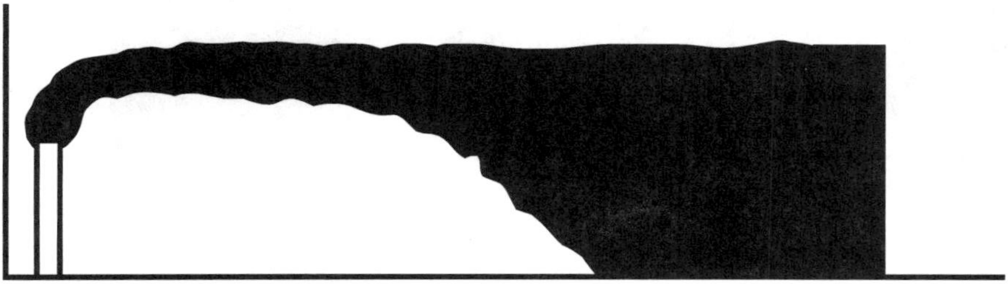

Figure 10.4. Inversion Breakup Dispersion Pattern.

10.3.3. Looping

This pattern is associated with sources that have relatively low heat emissions and short stacks. It is usually observed on warm days with clear skies and low-to-moderate wind speeds. The vertical temperature structure is usually unstable, creating large thermally induced eddies which bring the plume to the surface near the emission source.

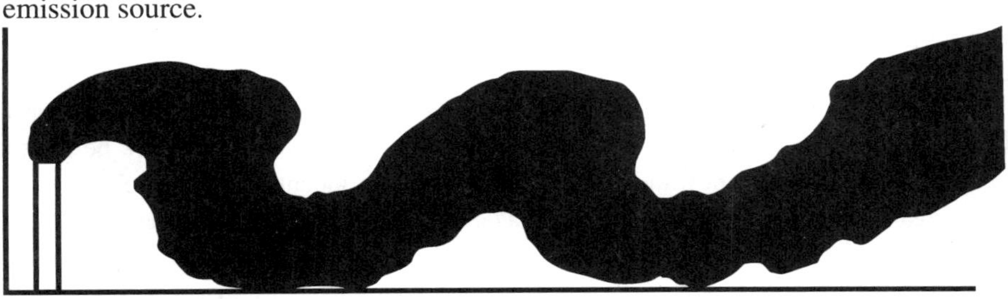

Figure 10.5. Looping Dispersion Pattern.

Surface concentrations associated with looping have short durations and sometimes exceed the levels of the more persistent surface concentrations experienced with the coning pattern.

10.3.4. Trapping or Capping Type Dispersion Limited Mixing Layer

The trapping dispersion pattern is also referred to as the limited mixing layer dispersion pattern. This pattern is important because the resulting maximum surface concentrations may be as much as three times that estimated under coning conditions. Maximum surface concentrations may persist for 2-4 hours, usually occurring from mid-morning to mid-afternoon.

Figure 10.6. Trapping Dispersion Pattern.

10.3.5. Relative Maximum Concentration Values for Dispersion Patterns

The value of maximum concentration due to any dispersion pattern depends on unit size, stack height and meteorological conditions. For early small units, the coning dispersion pattern occurs more frequently than other patterns. As a result, the maximum concentration due to the coning pattern was considered as the critical plume dispersion pattern.

With the increase in unit sizes there has been a increase in the height of stacks and therefore the plume dispersion pattern, which results in maximum concentration, has also changed. The magnitude of maximum surface concentrations from the coning pattern decreased, and the magnitude (relative to the coning pattern) of concentrations from the inversion breakup pattern increased.

However, the trapping pattern became more prominent for larger units with higher stacks and by the time unit size had increased to 900 MW and stack height to about 245 m, the frequency and magnitude of surface concentrations associated with trapping dispersion had increased to such a degree that this pattern became the critical pattern identified with plants of this size.

Although the magnitude of surface SO_2 concentrations is important, it alone does not necessarily establish the criticality of a particular plume dispersion pattern. The frequency of occurrence of a pattern and duration of the resulting concentrations must also be considered. Thus, for a particular power plant, a pattern resulting in maximum surface concentrations once or twice a year may be considered less critical than another which induces some lower concentrations 10 to 20 times a year.

10.3.6. Potential use of CNN as Plume Pattern Classifier

Two field methods for characterizing the rise and dispersion of plumes from tall chimneys are presented in Reference 6. Plume samples and meteorological data can be obtained from instruments on board aircraft to determine plume direction of travel, horizontal dispersion coefficients, rise, and emission fluxes. Photography of visible plumes can provide data on plume rise and vertical width, if orientation and scale are known. Aerial and ground-based photography were used to study plumes from a power station and copper smelter in Australia.

It is clear that the features of plumes and associated meteorological data can be used to drive a computational neural network that acts as a classifier to determine plume dispersion patterns. The result enables the next step of choosing the appropriate dispersion model for the pattern identified.

10.4. Plume Dispersion Models

Most work on environmental power dispatch has used the steady state pollution dispersion model, which is based on the assumption that the emission from a stack, during coning dispersion conditions, can be described by the Gaussian Plume Model (GPM) in the downwind and crosswind directions. The model was developed by Pasquill and Meade,[7] Turner,[8] and is derived in Viegell and Head[9] as a solution to the turbulent diffusion equation of a non-reacting pollutant in the atmosphere.

With steady state wind speed and direction, the pollutant concentration can be expressed in terms of source emission, field, and meteorological parameters:

$$X(x,y,z) = \frac{Q}{\pi\sigma_y\sigma_z\bar{u}}\exp\left(-\frac{1}{2}\left(\frac{h^2}{\sigma_z^2}+\frac{y^2}{\sigma_y^2}\right)\right) \tag{10.1}$$

where:

X	=	ground level concentration (μg/m^3)
Q	=	release rate of steady emissions of pollutant (μg/s)
h	=	effective source height (m)
x	=	downwind distance
y	=	crosswind distance
z	=	vertical distance

σ_y = crosswind plume standard deviation of the distribution (m)
σ_z = vertical plume standard deviation of the distribution (m)
$\bar{u}$ = mean wind speed (m/s) at h

The coning dispersion parameters, σ_y and σ_z are functions of the distance from the source, x, and atmospheric stability $\frac{\Delta\theta}{\Delta z}$.

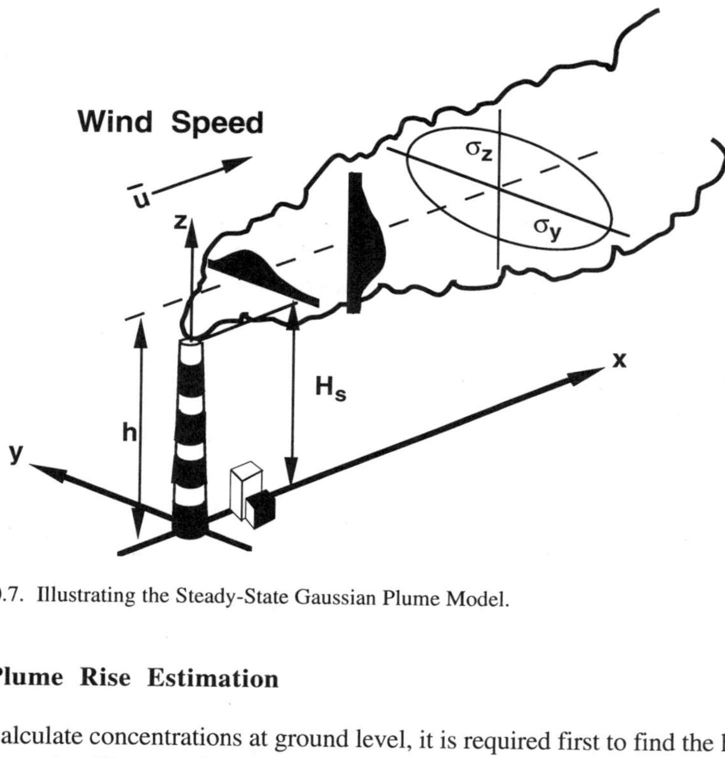

Figure 10.7. Illustrating the Steady-State Gaussian Plume Model.

10.5. Plume Rise Estimation

To calculate concentrations at ground level, it is required first to find the height to which a stack effluent will rise in the atmosphere. Much ambiguity exists with respect to the numerous formulae postulated to approximate the effective plume height for defined meteorological and operational conditions. The elevation of effective stack height, H_e, is the sum of the actual height of the stack, H_s, and of the plume rise, Δh.[10] A number of models of plume rise exist, the most commonly cited is the "2/3 Power Law."

10.5.1. 2/3 Plume Rise Model

The "2/3 Power Law" relation for calculating Δh is given by:

$$\Delta h = CF^{1/3}\overline{u}^{-1}x^{2/3} \qquad (10.2)$$

where:

$\overline{u}$ = The average wind speed between stack top and plume top,
x = horizontal downwind distance from stack.
C = a stability factor calculated using Eq. (10.1):

$$C = 1.065 - 6.25\left(\frac{\Delta\theta}{\Delta z}\right)\frac{m}{^\circ C} \qquad (10.3)$$

with:

$\frac{\Delta\theta}{\Delta z}$ = Average potential temperature gradient with height in °C/ 100 m
F = is the flux due to buoyancy and momentum, expressed as:

$$F = gV_s r^2 \frac{(\Delta T)}{T} \qquad (10.4)$$

with:

g = Acceleration due to gravity = 9.81 m/sec^2
r = Stack exit radius (m)
T = Ambient air temperature (K)
ΔT = Temperature difference between stack gas and ambient air (K)
V_s = Stack gas exit velocity (m/sec)

It is noted that the wind speed and heat emission rate are the principal determinants in calculating plume rise. The 2/3 power law formula embodies the principal quantities normally associated with the plume rise and permits some accounting for up to 15% difference in plume rise attributable to variation in atmospheric stability.

10.6. The NN Model

Our studies begin with the most popular neural network classifier, the multilayer perceptron (MLP),[11-12] with a continuous sigmoidal activation function. We use the back-propagation training algorithm with a momentum term α. We note that the success of the proposed network depends on careful consideration of the following aspects:

- Selection of the initial weights.
- Choice of scale factor η, steepness of the activation function λ, and momentum term α.

- Choice of architecture versus data representation.
- Network size, number of hidden layers, pruning and growth of the network.[13-14]

For example in Reference 14, it is shown that networks with one hidden layer perform better than those with two hidden layers. Further, a lower bound on the number of nodes in the hidden layer is derived and found to be d+1, where d is the dimension of the data patterns. The optimal number of nodes is shown to be somewhat larger than this (approximately 3d). In addition the network performance is shown to be relatively insensitive to overspecification of the network size. Finally it is shown that for near-optimal performance the number of training samples should be approximately 60d (d+1).

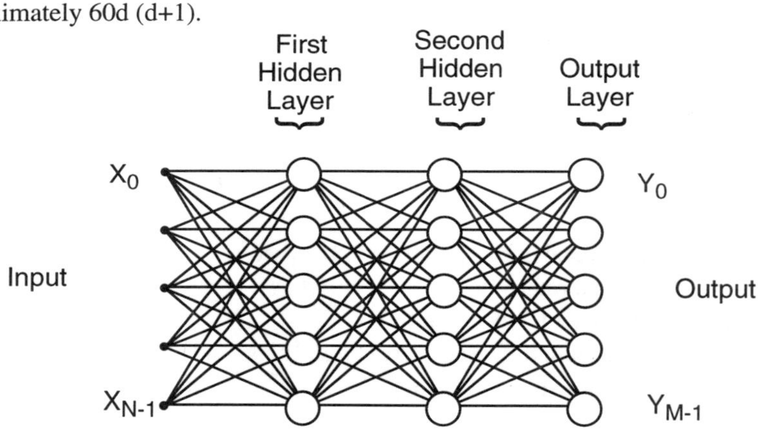

Figure 10.8. A Multi-layer Perceptron Neural Network.

10.7. Synthetic Plume Height Experiment

10.7.1. Typical Plume Height Model Data

Typical values cited in Reference 10 are as follows:

Stack height H_s (m)	182.9	152.4	76.2	121.9	91.4	152.4
Stack diameter (m)	7.9	7.6	4.3	4.3	5.0	6.3

In addition:

$\bar{u}$ = 1.0 - 16.8 m/sec (average wind speed between stack top and plume top)

x = 1219 m (horizontal downwind distance from stack)

Representative values of C given in Reference 10 are:

Class 1 $C = 1.07$ Inversion $\frac{\Delta\theta}{\Delta z} > 1$

Class 2 $C = 1.04$ Stable $0 < \frac{\Delta\theta}{\Delta z} < 1$

Class 3 $C = 0.98$ Neutral and unstable $\frac{\Delta\theta}{\Delta z} < 0$

with the range:

$\frac{\Delta\theta}{\Delta z}$ -0.53 to -3.74 °C $(100\ \text{m})^{-1}$

r = stack exit radius (m)

T = ambient air temperature = 273 - 304 °K

T_s = stack gas temperature 106-145 °C (convert to K by adding 273.15)

ΔT = temp. difference between stack gas and ambient air (K)

V_S = stack gas exit velocity = 7.7 - 29.2 m/sec

Table 10.1: Vertical potential temperature gradients[5]

Condition	**Temperature Gradient** $(\frac{\Delta\theta}{\Delta z})$
Neutral	0.00
Slightly stable	0.27
Stable	0.64
Isothermal	1.00
Moderate inversion	1.36
Strong inversion	1.73

10.7.2. Numerical Example

$\frac{\Delta\theta}{\Delta z}$ = 1.73

$\bar{u}$ = 8.5 m/sec

x = 1219 m

ΔT = 120 (K)

V_S = 15.6 m/sec

T = 291 (K)

Calculates F = 984.64 $\text{m}^4\ \text{sec}^{-3}$

C = 0.96

As a result:

$\Delta h = 114\, C\, F\, (1/3)\, u^{-1} = 128$ m

10.7.3. Observed Plume Rise Data

Table 10.2: Observed Plume Rise Data

Stability Class	Wind Speed C	Observed Plume Rise, y	2/3 Power Law, yc
2	1.9	331	645
2	3.3	363	374
2	3.4	457	354
2	3.7	363	323
2	4.1	295	298
2	4.5	329	266
2	4.7	195	255
2	5.2	308	249
2	5.2	182	266
2	6.0	188	194
2	7.7	219	156
2	8.0	191	172
2	8.4	154	158
2	10.0	94	134
2	10.6	165	127
2	10.8	110	125
2	11.4	135	106
2	13.8	150	96
2	2.1	555	528
2	2.1	476	526
2	2.2	460	506
2	2.5	303	447
2	2.5	347	442
2	2.8	312	389
2	2.9	317	383
2	3.1	250	396
2	3.2	251	335
2	4.6	259	252
2	5.0	207	230
2	5.0	220	220
2	5.1	226	216
2	5.2	359	219
2	5.4	208	211
2	5.8	215	197
2	5.9	165	190
2	6.9	180	162
2	10.4	165	110
2	2.2	333	520
2	2.4	316	492
2	3.4	304	337
2	4.1	301	290
2	4.8	155	243
2	5.2	138	231
2	6.5	136	181

10.7.4. Preliminary Test Results

For the set of observed plume rise data, we tested a number of proposed neural network configurations with two hidden layers. In each case, we selected $H_1 = 20$ and $H_2 = 2$. The momentum term is taken as $\alpha = 0.9$, with the following error results in Table 10.3.

Table 10.3: Error Results

η	SSE
0.7	0.0312
0.5	0.0297
0.3	0.031

*Each case was allowed to run for 1,500,000 iterations.

10.8. Synthetic Coning Dispersion Data

10.8.1. Typical Data for Coning Dispersion Model

Our initial experiments are based on training using and then predicting the ratio of X to Q for situations associated with characteristics given in Carpenter *et. al.*[5] shown in Figures 10.9 and 10.10.

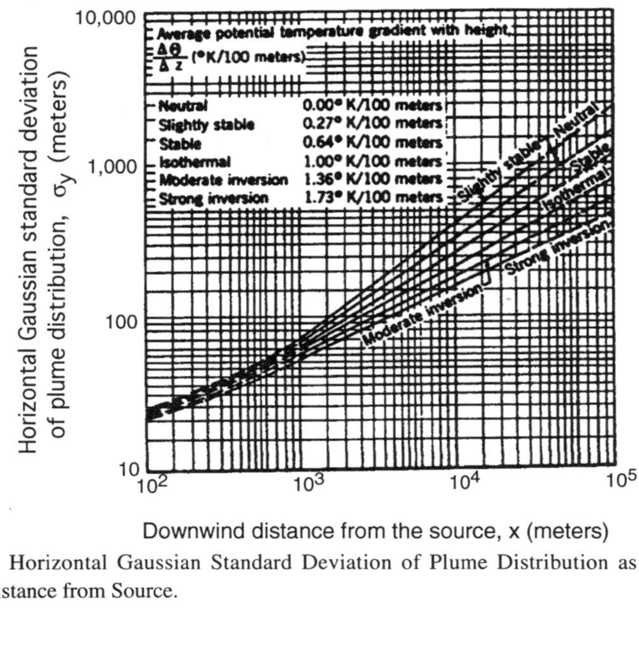

Figure 10.9. Horizontal Gaussian Standard Deviation of Plume Distribution as a Function of Downwind Distance from Source.

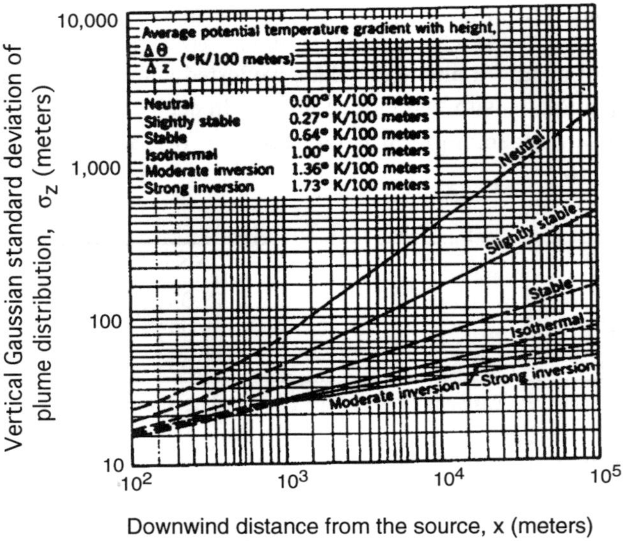

Figure 10.10. Vertical Gaussian Standard Deviation of Plume Distribution as a Function of Downwind Distance from Source.

10.8.2. Coning Dispersion Model Test Data:

Initial tests are conducted using the coning dispersion model for h = 150m with $\sigma_y = \sigma_z = 200$ m. The resulting model has two independent variables U and y. For our experiments, we vary U from 2 to 10 in steps of 0.5 m/s and y from 200 to 2000 in steps of 100, for training. We use the trained network to predict the output for U from 2.1 in steps of 0.5 and y from 250 m in steps of 100.

10.9. References

1. Y.V. Orlov, I.G. Persiantsev and S.P. Rebrik, "Application of neural networks to fluorescent diagnostics of organic pollution in natural waters," in *Proceedings 1993 IEEE International Conference on Neural Networks* (San Francisco, CA, 28 March - 1 April 1993), vol. 3, pp. 1230-1235.
2. T. Albrecht, G. Matz, T. Hunte and J. Hildemann, "An intelligent gas sensor system for the identification of hazardous airborne compounds using an array of semiconductor gas sensors and Kohonen feature map neural networks," *Second International Conference on 'Intelligent Systems Engineering,'* IEE Conf. Publ. No. 395, (Hamburg-Harburg, Germany, 5-9 Sept. 1994), pp. 130-137.

3. D.C. Park, *et. al.*, "Electric Load Forecasting Using an Artificial Neural Network," *IEEE Transactions on Power Systems* **6** (1991) 442-449.
4. T.D. King, M.E. El-Hawary, and Ferial El-Hawary, "Optimal Environmental Dispatching of Electric Power Systems Via an Improved Hopfield Neural Network," Accepted for publication in *IEEE Transactions on Power Systems* and the *1995 Winter Power Meeting* (New York, February 1995).
5. S.B. Carpenter, T.L. Montgomery, J.M. Leavitt, W.C. Colbaugh and F.W. Thomas, "Principal Plume Dispersion Models. TVA Power Plants," *Journal of the Air Pollution Control Association* **21** (1971) 491-495.
6. N. Carras, and D.J. Williams, "Description of Plume and Pollution Measurement Using Aircraft and Photography," *Air Pollution Problems & Model Workshop* (Cape Schanck, Australia, 1993) and *Clean Air-Australia* **27(4)** (November 1993) p. 206.
7. F. Pasquill and P.J. Meade, "A Study of the Average Distribution of Pollution around Staythoope," *Int. J. Air Poll.* **1** (1958) 60.
8. D.B. Turner, "A Diffusion Model for an Urban Area," *J. Applied Meteorology* **3** (1964) 83.
9. W.J. Viegell and J.H. Head, "Derivation of the Gaussian Plume Model," *JAPCA* **28** (1978) 1139-1141.
10. F.W. Thomas, S.B. Carpenter and W.C. Colbaugh, "Plume Rise Estimates for Electric Generating Stations," *Journal of the Air Pollution Control Association* **20** (1970) 170-177.
11. Jacek M. Zurada, *Introduction to Artificial Neural Systems* (West Publishing Co., 1992).
12. Simon Haykin, *Neural Networks, A Comprehensive Foundation* (IEEE Press, Piscataway, NJ, 1994).
13. R. Reed, "Pruning Algorithms-A Survey," *IEEE Transactions on Neural Networks* **4** (1993) 740-747.
14. D.R. Hush, "Classification with neural networks: a performance analysis," *IEEE International Conference on Systems Engineering* (IEEE, Piscataway, NJ, 1989), pp. 277-80.

11. INVESTIGATION OF NEURAL-NET BASED CONTROL STRATEGIES FOR IMPROVED POWER SYSTEM DYNAMIC PERFORMANCE

DEJAN J. SOBAJIC
Electric Power Research Institute, 3412 Hillview Avenue
Palo Alto, California 94304-1395, USA
E-mail: dsobajic@msm.epri.com

ABSTRACT

The ability to accurately predict the behavior of a dynamic system is of essential importance in monitoring and control of complex processes. In this regard recent advances in neural-net based system identification represent a significant step toward development and design of a new generation of control tools for increased system performance and reliability. The enabling functionality is the one of accurate representation of a model of a nonlinear and nonstationary dynamic system. This functionality provides valuable new opportunities including:

1. The ability to predict future system behavior on the basis of actual system observations,
2. On-line evaluation and display of system performance and design of early warning systems, and
3. Controller optimization for improved system performance.

In this presentation, we discuss the issues involved in definition and design of learning control systems and their impact on power system control. Several numerical examples are provided for illustrative purpose.

12. FEASIBILITY OF USING ADAPTIVE LOGIC NETWORKS TO PREDICT COMPRESSOR UNIT FAILURE

WILLIAM W. ARMSTRONG, PH.D.
Dendronic Decisions Limited, 3624 - 108 Street, NW
Edmonton, Alberta, Canada T6J 1B4
E-mail: arms@cs.ualberta.ca

and

Department of Computing Science, University of Alberta
Edmonton, Alberta, Canada T6G 2H1

CHUNGYING CHU, M.SC.
Dendronic Decisions Limited, 3624 - 108 Street, NW
Edmonton, Alberta, Canada T6J 1B4

and

MONROE M. THOMAS, B.SC.
Department of Computing Science, University of Alberta
Edmonton, Alberta, Canada T6G 2H1

ABSTRACT

In this feasibility study, an adaptive logic network (ALN) was trained to predict failures of turbine-driven compressor units using a large database of measurements. No expert knowledge about compressor systems was involved. The predictions used only the statistical properties of the measurements and the indications of failure types. A fuzzy set was used to model measurements typical of normal operation. It was constrained by a requirement, imposed during ALN training, that it should have a shape similar to a Gaussian density, more precisely, that its logarithm should be convex-up. Initial results obtained using this approach to knowledge discovery in the database were encouraging.
Keywords: knowledge discovery, data mining, adaptive logic network, ALN, neural network, prediction.

12.1. Introduction

The company for which this study was done maintains a database of sensor measurements from various compressor unit components recorded at regular intervals. The database also contains the dates and times that each compressor unit was started and stopped, and the reason for each stoppage. The number of measurements made on each unit in each interval is quite large (around 130) so, given this wealth of data, some automated method of determining a unit's health based on these measurements was thought to be feasible. It was felt that savings could be realized in the maintenance of compressor stations if a predictive maintenance strategy were used instead of a run-to-failure or scheduled-maintenance strategy. The savings achieved would be greatest if the prediction methods were very accurate, and could predict failure several hours or even days in advance.

The prediction method discussed here is applicable not only to compressors, but to many situations where data monitoring some process is continuously collected. It is a technique for doing what has been called "knowledge discovery" or "data mining". Companies are creating "data warehouses" for the purpose of filtering, summarizing and archiving data that they collect during their operations so the data are available in a homogeneous format for subsequent analysis and decision-making. Many tools developed in the area of artificial intelligence have been used to analyze data, including rule induction and machine learning paradigms.[1] Adaptive Logic Networks (ALNs) are used in the present study to analyze compressor data. Their other areas of application include particle physics,[2] rehabilitation of persons with spinal cord injury[3-5] and real-time control of mechanical systems.[6]

12.2. Adaptive Logic Networks

The ALN discussed in this paper is a type of feedforward multilayer perceptron which uses linear threshold units in a first hidden layer, and logic gates AND and OR in other hidden layers and in the output layer. The units form a tree with a single Boolean output. ALNs cannot output analog values directly, so in that case, the goal is to get the net to produce a 1 output for points *on and under the graph of a function*, and a 0 otherwise, as suggested in Figure 12.1.

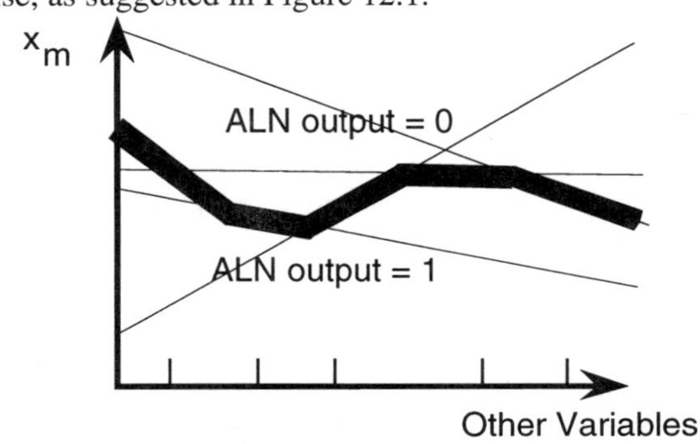

Figure 12.1. How an ALN represents a function.

ALNs *implicitly* represent piecewise linear functions. Linear functions L_i: $x_m = w_{i,0} + w_{i,1}x_1 + \ldots + w_{i,m-1}x_{m-1}$ (shown as thin lines in Figure 12.1) are joined using a tree expression of MAXIMUM and MINIMUM operations (corresponding to the OR and AND units in the ALN tree) to form a piecewise linear function: $x_m =$

$f(x_1,\ldots,x_m)$ (shown as the thick curve in Figure 12.1). Each linear piece L_i in a trained ALN can be thought of as the being learned by least squares fitting (or linear regression) on the data points in a certain portion of the input space. L_i is required to fit a data point $(x_1,\ldots,x_{m-1})$ if for the given values of the first m - 1 components, L_i is the piece determining the value of f according to the MAX/MIN expression. It is the *active* linear piece in the function graph for that input.

Like other supervised networks, ALNs learn functions from empirical data presented to them during a phase called *training*. In training, the ALN does least squares fitting using many linear pieces at once. The difference between this ALN adaptation algorithm and many separate least squares procedures running in parallel is this: as linear pieces shift during training, they each gain or lose points of the training set according to which piece is active for a given training point, so the problem is always changing for each individual linear piece.

After training, a decision tree (DTREE) is created that partitions the (m-1)-dimensional input space into blocks, in each of which the function is represented by a simple expression containing a few linear pieces connected by MAXIMUM and MINIMUM operations. (Dividing the horizontal axis in Figure 12.1 near midpoints of the thick line segments results in intervals B_k, each involving one or two linear pieces only.) Each such expression is much smaller than the expression representing the whole ALN. By not having to do all the arithmetic operations to evaluate all linear functions, the decision tree approach makes evaluation of each individual output very fast and efficient. The "open architecture" of DTREE evaluation also allows scrutiny of the learned function in a way not possible with other multilayer neural networks, unless they are shallow or have few nodes. Examination of DTREEs has been used in our study to determine the important variables for predicting specific types of compressor unit failure. In other cases, the DTREE can be used to check that the net will not give any unexpected outputs.

Most neural nets do not allow convenient use of human expertise, which is particularly unfortunate if there is some guidance that an expert could provide about the function being learned – some of its qualitative properties, say. In the present study, no expert knowledge was used, but an *ad hoc* assumption was made that the function of the measurements representing normalcy of operation of the compressor was unimodal and had a simple shape. By choosing the network architecture of an ALN and restricting values of weights during training, the desired shape could be achieved.

Further details of use of the above type of ALN may be found in Reference 6 The program used in this study was Atree 3.0 beta release 2, a commercial product being developed by Dendronic Decisions Limited. An Atree 3.0 demonstration program that runs under Windows 3.x on the IBM® PC and compatibles and that has considerable on-line documentation can be obtained electronically.[7]

12.3. Finding Possible Predictors of Failure

In order to determine if there is a possible indication of failure contained in the measurements of any individual parameter, a statistical analysis was performed on all parameters to (1) determine whether a failure of any (unspecified) type could be predicted from the chosen parameter, and (2) determine whether a failure of a specific subsystem could be predicted from the chosen parameter. There was not enough data present for the single compressor station targeted to do these studies for all possible types of failure.

For failure runs, the mean and standard deviation of each parameter were calculated for the first 50% of the run, and then again for the last six hours of the run. The ratio of the absolute value of the difference in means of the two sets to the standard deviation of the normal set was used as an indicator of the relative importance of the parameter in detecting a change to the failure state from the normal state.

Table 12.1 gives the idea of some of the measurements and their analyses (actually there were close to 200 parameters measured or derived). The meanings of the columns in the tables are as follows:

Parameter: The number of the parameter.
MeanNorm: The mean value of the parameter in the normal set.
DevNorm: The standard deviation of the parameter in the normal set.
MeanFail: The mean value of the parameter within the last six hours before the failure event.
| MeanNorm - MeanFail | /DevNorm: Relative deviation in the means of the parameter.

It can be seen that parameter 14 is likely to be more significant for prediction of failure than parameter 12. No parameter (except for one with an anomaly) showed a relative deviation in means beyond 1.0, so the conclusion from this analysis was that "no single parameter could reliably predict general unit failure."

A more careful analysis of *subsystem specific* failure was carried out as before. Again, "no single parameter showed itself useful as a predictor of any of the subsystem failure types examined."

Although analysis revealed that no single parameter can be used to reliably predict unit failure, taking the parameters with the greatest ratios **|(MeanNorm - MeanFail)| / DevNorm** was conjectured to be likely to pick out a useful subset of parameters for study using ALN prediction. Twenty variables with the largest ratios were chosen for further analysis. This is certainly not the best set possible. Although one of the parameters with a large ratio had been shown to be irrelevant for predicting failure, it was included as a training parameter to verify that an ALN can learn to ignore unimportant variables.

Table 12.1: Parameter statistics for all failure types (truncated)

Parameter	MeanNorm	DevNorm	MeanFail	| MeanNorm - MeanFail | / DevNorm
1	0.661642	0.10828	0.64987	0.108717
2	9.68249	26.6494	7.06494	0.098222
3	88.5379	1.35222	88.474	0.0472354
4	2.61525	12.0579	1.66883	0.07849
5	18.4023	5.40602	18.987	0.108153
6	987.459	390.765	1041.08	0.137215
7	620.693	82.311	630.078	0.114013
8	6110.59	391.197	6153.19	0.108919
9	0.543992	0.211078	0.55026	0.0296929
10	44.7623	7.13785	44.0584	0.0986141
11	24.5751	0.822201	24.6494	0.0903105
12	25.8062	0.667883	25.7922	0.0209886
13	21.2	1.18058	21.013	0.158408
14	4528.33	456.669	4427.29	0.221271
15	5726.8	219.124	5685.77	0.187281

12.4. Setting Up Training and Test Sets

Training sets were built using two parts extracted from all the failure runs that lasted longer than a fixed minimum duration. The measurements from first the 50% of each such run were deemed to indicate that the unit was running in a normal state. This data is called the *normal set.* The measurements from the last six hours of the run (before failure shutdown) are deemed to indicate that the unit is in a failure state. That set is called the *failure set.* The test sets were composed of all the failure runs. During testing, the ALN evaluates considerable data it has not seen during training, however the first half of the training runs as well as the last six hours of training runs must be excluded in attempting to measure generalization.

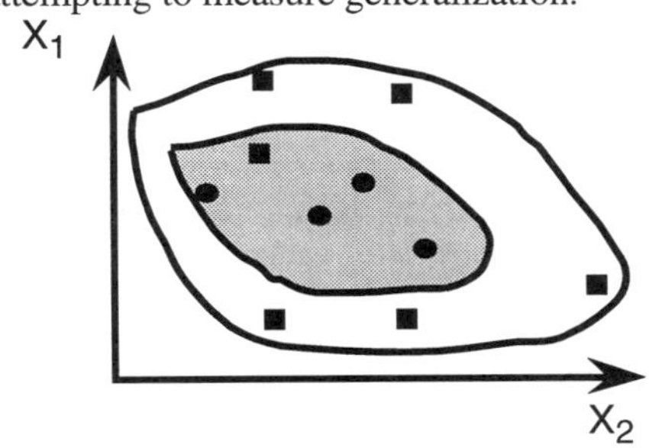

Figure 12.2. Normal operation in shaded area.

Using the twenty parameters $(x_0,x_1,\ldots,x_{19})$ and the normal/failure classification, a training set for a function $x_{20} = N(x_0,x_1,\ldots,x_{19})$ could be generated as follows. The desired output x_{20} would be set to 1 in a training sample if the unit is in a normal state. The other measurement vectors would be associated with a certain x_{20} value close to 0. If there were just two parameters x_0 and x_1, then a normal set might look like the black dots in the shaded part of Figure 12.2. During normal operation, the compressor's measurements should usually stay within the shaded region. The second curve, outside the boundary of the shaded part, is such that outside of it, the compressor is in a "failure" state requiring shutdown and repair or adjustment. The area outside the shaded part but inside the other curve is an area of uncertainty about the health of the compressor. Several black squares are intended to indicate measurements in the failure set, made just before shutdown.

To indicate the degree to which any possible vector of measurements $(x_0,x_1,\ldots,x_{19})$ indicates normal behavior, we used the *fuzzy set concept.* The "fuzzy set" N ("normal") is a function which has the following properties:

- the value of N on points of the shaded region is close to 1
- the value of N outside the outer curve is close to 0
- the value of N between the two curves is in the interval [0,1] and tends to increase as a measurement vector gets closer to the shaded region.

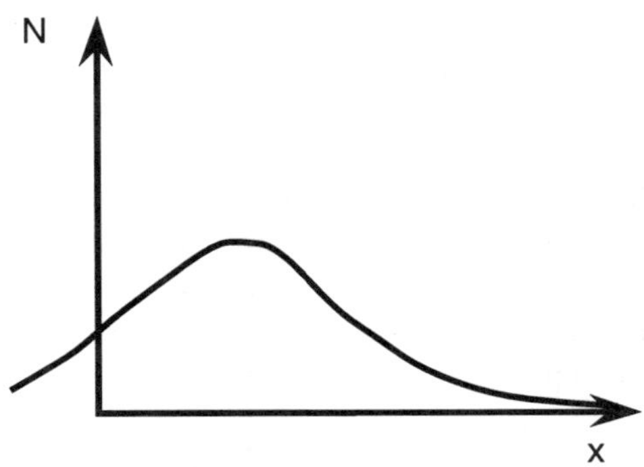

Figure 12.3. Fuzzy set "normal operation."

In order to use ALNs effectively by taking advantage of the possibility of specifying qualitative properties of a function, we didn't try to learn the fuzzy set N directly, but rather the value of ln N. To motivate this we consider the situation if normal operation was guaranteed at only one point, and the uncertainly about normalcy of a measurement varied somewhat like a Gaussian density. Then, looked at from the side, our function N would appear as in Figure 12.3.

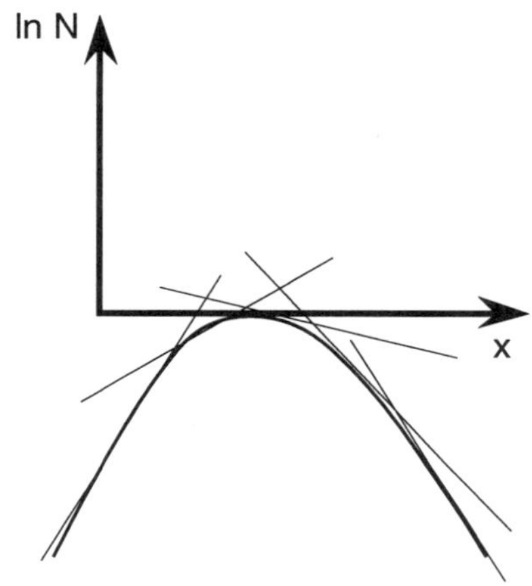

Figure 12.4. Fitting the natural logarithm of the fuzzy set with linear pieces.

The natural logarithm of N is shown in Figure 12.4. It is a convex set. In the case of the Gaussian (for a single random variate) the density has the form $N = \frac{1}{\sqrt{2\pi\sigma}} e^{-\frac{x^2}{2\sigma^2}}$, and the logarithm has the form $\ln N = \ln\left(\frac{1}{\sqrt{2\pi\sigma}}\right) - \frac{x^2}{2\sigma^2}$. The latter is the equation of a parabola. Passing to the logarithm of N can thus simplify the of the shape of the curve by removing the inflection points and making it easy to approximate by linear pieces. The thin lines in Figure 12.4 show several linear pieces fitting the parabola.

The situation in higher dimensions is similar. The logarithm of the Gaussian density is a paraboloid, and the surface can be fitted with high-dimensional planes using as structure of an ALN just one AND node. The density functions whose logarithm is convex form a larger set than the class of Gaussian distributions; we refer to them as the "log-convex" distributions. We know of no other studies using this class.

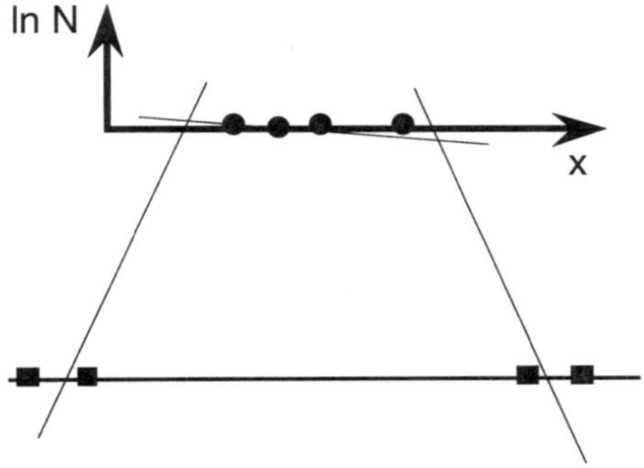

Figure 12.5. Approximating a convex surface with an AND of three linear pieces.

The *ad hoc* assumption that the uncertainty about the health of a compressor can be captured by a log-convex fuzzy set was used to set up an ALN. The training set described above was replaced by one that had the values of the natural logarithm of x_{20} in place of x_{20}. The thin lines of Figure 12.5 approximate a convex surface with a plateau. At the top of the plateau are the known normal-running measurements, while further down are the measurements close to shutdown. They are represented by the dark squares. The level of the horizontal line they are placed on is unimportant, since that merely changes the task to be learned by the ALN by a constant scale factor. It was decided to use a shutdown level of -10, corresponding to a fuzzy membership of the points in the normal set of $e^{-10} = 0.000045$.

12.5. Training the ALN and Testing Generalization

Using this training set, an ALN was trained to have a final root mean square error on the training set of about 1.0. When used to classify input points, it generated a classification value in the range [-10, 0], which indicates the natural log of the membership in the normal set. A threshold of -2 corresponding to a fuzzy set membership of $e^{-2} = 0.1353$ was chosen so that an ALN output in the range [-10, -2] was classified as being in the failure set, and an ALN output in the range (-2, 0] was classified as being in the normal set. Using this threshold, the trained ALN correctly classified 83.1% of the failure set points and 99.6% of the normal set points in the *training* set.

To test *generalization* of the trained ALN, it is presented with portions of the failure runs not seen during training. Table 12.2 illustrates a trend to classify the points closer to the end of a failure run as being in the failure set and shows that the ALN has a tendency to correctly predict failure.

Table 12.2: Testing Generalization of the Trained ALN

% of failure run duration	**50-60**	**60-70**	**70-80**	**80-90**	**90-100**
proportion classified as failure	0.13	0.26	0.28	0.33	0.52
proportion classified as normal	0.86	0.73	0.71	0.66	0.47

The last six hours of readings, only two or three points per run, contained in the "90-100% of failure run duration" category, were present during training. Hence the right-hand column is not an entirely valid test of ALN generalization, but the other columns are. The results in Table 12.2 reveal an important ability of the trained ALN: in some cases it started to predict failure well before shutdown of the compressor.

12.6. Predicting the Failure Type

In a complex system like a compressor station, predicting that a failure is likely to occur is much more useful if accompanied by some indication of what kind of failure may be. The results indicated that the ALN can sometimes predict the type of failure. After an ALN is trained, it can be converted to a human readable DTREE format. When a DTREE is used to evaluate an input point, the program indicates the linear piece that was used to calculate the value of the function. For example, when the DTREE derived from the trained ALN in this study calculates a value less than -2.0 (indicating failure) for the failure runs of a specific type, say X, the value was always calculated from one of the linear pieces indexed 4, 9, 11, or 21. With another failure type, Y, the linear pieces indexed 19 and 15 were responsible for predicting failure. Hence the linear pieces seemed be providing useful information about the failure type. The weights on these pieces are important in connecting a failure type to variables which are important for predicting it.

12.7. Temporal Behavior of the Predictor

Figure 12.6 shows how the performance measure learned by the ALN declines before a failure shutdown. *Note that time within a run advances to the left.* Low values at the left indicate a prediction of breakdown. These are a selection of "good" examples, though in one case the prediction of failure seems, to say the least, premature. There were also examples where the prediction was quite wrong.

12.8. Conclusion

The conclusion of this feasibility study, mainly derived from Table 12.2, is that ALNs show some promise in predicting compressor failures several hours, sometimes days, in advance of the actual shutdown time. Analysis of the fuzzy set indicating normalcy of operation suggested that one may even be able to predict the failure type by noting which linear piece is active for the measurement vectors obtained from the compressor system before failure.

A more comprehensive study incorporating expert knowledge of the compressor system could be expected to lead to more accurate predictions. In particular, further analyses of the piecewise linear functions produced by an ALN would reveal the most useful combinations of measurements for predicting specific failure types. We emphasize that the above results are preliminary, and this paper is intended only to illustrate an approach to predictive maintenance using ALNs.

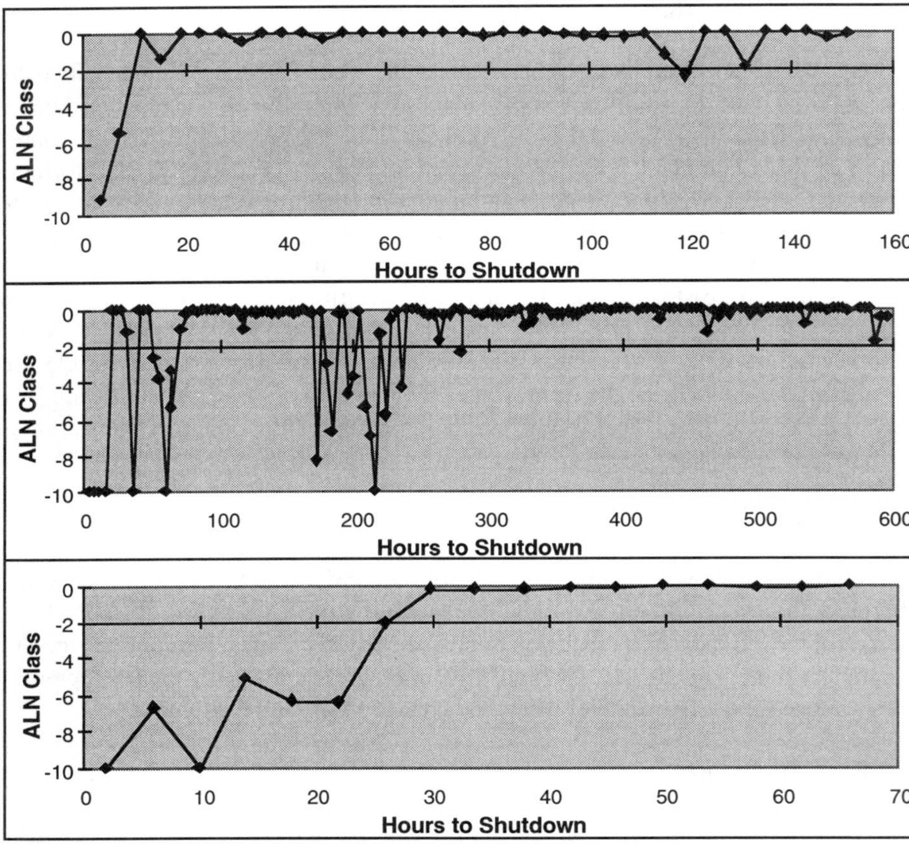

Figure 12.6 This figure graphs how the performance measure learned by the ALN declines before a failure shutdown.

12.9. References

1. Gregory Piatetsky-Shapiro and William J. Frawley eds., *Knowledge Discovery in Databases* (MIT Press, Cambridge, MA, 1991), ISBN 0-262-66070-9.
2. Stefan C. Kremer and Stan Melax, "Using Adaptive Logic Networks for Quick Recognition of Particles," *1994 IEEE International Conf. on Neural Networks* vol. 5 (Orlando, Florida, June 27 - 29, 1994), pp. 3015-3019.
3. D.B. Popovic, R.B. Stein, K.L. Jovanovic, R. Dai, A. Kostov, W.W. Armstrong, "Sensory Nerve Recording for Closed-Loop Control to Restore Motor Functions," *IEEE Trans. Biomed. Eng.* **40** (1993) 1024-1031.

4. Aleksandar Kostov, Richard B. Stein, Dejan Popovic and W.W. Armstrong, "Improved Methods for Control of FES for Locomotion," in *Proc. International Federation of Automatic Control (IFAC) Symposium on Modeling and Control in Biomedical Systems* (Galveston, Texas, USA, March 27 - 30, 1994).
5. William W. Armstrong, Aleksandar Kostov, Richard B. Stein and Monroe M. Thomas, "Adaptive Logic Networks in Rehabilitation," *Workshop on Environmental and Energy Applications of Neural Networks* (Battelle Pacific National Laboratories, Richland, WA, March 30 - 31, 1995).
6. William W. Armstrong and Monroe M. Thomas, "Control of a vehicle active suspension system using adaptive logic networks," in *WCNN '94 Program Addendum*, (International Neural Network Society, Washington, DC, 1994) pp. 9-14. This is available in the Internet from ftp.cs.ualberta.ca in file pub/atree/wcnnpub.ps.Z (compressed PostScript® format).
7. Monroe M. Thomas and William W. Armstrong, Atree 3.0 Demo in pub/atree/aln3demo.zip via FTP from ftp.cs.ualberta.ca. It is also available on CompuServe ("GO DENDRONIC").

13. NEAR AND LONG-TERM LOAD PREDICTION USING RADIAL BASIS FUNCTION NETWORKS

MONTE F. HANCOCK, JR., M.S.
Computer Science Innovations (CSI), Inc., 1235 Evans Road
Melbourne, Florida 32904-2314, USA
E-mail: mhancock@csihq.com

and

Department of Mathematics and Computer Science, Rollins College
Winter Park, Florida, USA

ABSTRACT

A number of researchers have investigated the application of multi-layer perceptrons (MLP's), a variety of neural network, to the problem of short-term load forecasting for electric utilities (e.g., Rahman & Hazin, IEEE Trans. Power Systems, May 1993). "Short-term" in this context typically means "next day." These forecasts have been based upon previous day actual loads and meteorological factors (e.g., max-min temperature, relative humidity).

We describe the application of radial basis function networks (RBF's) to the "long-term" (next year) load forecasting problem. The RBF network performs a two-stage classification based upon annual average loads and meteorological data. During stage 1, discrete classification is performed using radius-limited elements. During stage 2, a multi-layer perceptron may be applied. The quantized output is used to correct a prediction template.

The stage 1 classifier is trained by maximizing an objective function (the "disambiguity"). The stage 2 MLP's are trained by standard back-propagation.

This work uses 12 months of hourly meteorological data, and the corresponding hourly load data for both commercial and residential feeders. At the current stage of development, the RBF machine can train on 20% of the weather/load data (selected by simple linear sampling), and estimate the hourly load for an entire year (8,760 data points) with 9.1% error (RMS, relative to daily peak load). (By comparison, monthly mean profiles perform at c. 12% error.) The best short-term load forecasters operate in the 2% error range. The current system is an engineering prototype, and development is continuing.

More significant than the present (modest) performance figures are the techniques being used for development. Of particular importance are:

The RBF paradigm and "safe interpolation"
Data coding and quantization
Taxonomic Decomposition

This research has been conducted under IR&D at Computer Science Innovations, Inc. (CSI), Melbourne, Florida from 1991-1995.

(Note: subsequent work has improved the reported results from 9.1% RMS error to under 3% RMS error.)

13.1. Technical Background / Nomenclature

13.1.1. Classification Problems

Classification is a special case of the general regression problem, for which the range of the regression function is a discrete set. Desired classification decisions are specified at exemplars, and extended throughout the problem domain by tuning the parameters of a decision function. Inputs to the classifier are usually M-dimensional vectors of "features", and the finitely many discrete outputs are the "classes." Given this understanding, many conventional statistical notions (e.g., RMS error, type 1/type 2 errors) apply.

13.1.2. Feature Space, Goal Space, and Parameter Space

The M-dimensional Euclidean space spanned by the vectors of features for a particular classification problem is called the problem's "feature space." Feature space is the domain of the decision function.

The decision function assigns to each feature vector a "class." The set of all classes is "goal space." Goal space is the range of the decision function; it is just a set, and has no topological or algebraic properties.

A decision function is an instantiation of a parameterized decision function model; let this model have L>0 tunable parameters. Each decision function, then, is represented by a point in L-dimensional Euclidean space. This space is called "parameter space." (For a trainable classifier, parameter space will be the domain of an "objective function", which measures the performance of the classifier.)

13.1.3. Trainable Classifiers

If training is understood to be "incremental improvement of performance through experience and self-adjustment", then trainable classifiers can be built.

We describe a typical variant of so-called "supervised "training (examples of known classification available).[1] The process is a closed-loop optimization (see Figure 13.1), during which a fixed collection of feature vectors (the "training set") is repeatedly presented to the classifier. After each cycle of presentations ("epoch"), the overall performance of the classifier is measured via an objective function. The parameters of the decision function are then adjusted in an attempt to increase the objective function's value on the next epoch.

Training can be regarded, then, as a search of parameter space for global maxima of the objective function with respect to the given training set. Standard optimization techniques may apply (e.g., gradient search, least squares, "filtering" techniques), and emerging techniques are the subject of current research (e.g., back propagation, simulated annealing, genetic algorithms, cascade correlation).[2]

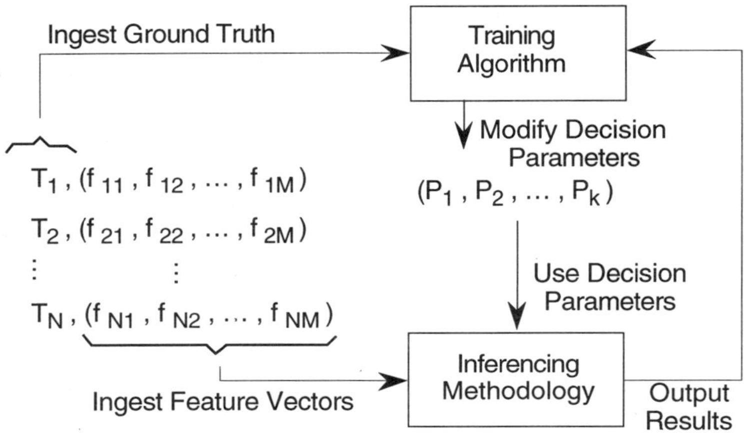

Figure 13.1. Learning by "Feedback and Adaptation."

13.2. RBF Networks: Brief Conceptual Tutorial

RBF's attack the regression problem in much the same way "partitions of unity" attack the spectral problem.[3] They operate in the feature space itself, exploiting its geometry to directly model clusters and their boundaries, using many local interpolators of compact support.

RBF's can be regarded as neural networks in the sense that they operate by aggregation of the outputs of many discrete units which are trained rather then programmed. In distinction to most other neural paradigms, however, the elements in an RBF do not communicate with each other.

13.2.1. Stage 1 of the RBF: The Basis Functions

Stage 1 of an RBF's is constructed by positioning at each exemplar in feature space a compactly-supported pseudo-metric. These "basis functions" can be viewed as locally conditioning feature space with a "belief" field, much as an electric charge conditions nearby space with an electric field.

An individual basis function establishes a field of belief that a point in its region of feature space is in the same class as the basis function's exemplar. This belief decreases as we move away from the exemplar, becoming zero at a finite distance. The basis functions are therefore referred to as "radius-limited elements."

To use the basis functions to classify a point in feature space, the outputs of the basis functions in whose support it lies are combined by superposition according to an aggregation rule. This gives a vector of beliefs, component j being the belief that the point is in class j. The largest vector component designates the stage 1 classification. The relative sizes of the beliefs can be used to form a stage 1 classification confidence.

13.2.2. Stage 2 of the RBF: The Perceptron

The stage 1 classification can be used as the RBF output. It is customary, however, to apply a multi-layer perceptron[4] using the original feature vector and its stage 1 belief vector as inputs. The output of the perceptron then becomes the RBF output. (The rationale for using stage 1 as a pre-processor for a perceptron is that the stage 1 procedures can eliminate non-separability, which is problematic for perceptrons.)

13.2.3. The Bayesian Classifier is "Almost" a Stage 1 RBF

The Bayesian classifier is seen to be very similar to a stage 1 radial basis function classifier, with each class represented by a single element located at the class mean, and having local pseudo-metrics given by weighted quadratic exponentials. The only difference is that the exponentials do not have compact support (though in all real implementations, they will have).

The general stage 1 RBF will have many elements representing each class, and possibly different pseudo-metrics. The level-sets of the pseudo-metric give the fundamental shapes being used to cover clusters in feature space.

13.2.4. Other Interpretations of RBF Classifiers

The stage 1 RBF may also be regarded as a spectral decomposition of the density function for the given classification problem. Properly speaking, of course, this is a spatial rather than spectral decomposition, and the basis functions constitute a frame rather than a basis. This is the sense in which the "partition of unity" analogy with RBF's is instructive.

It is possible at this point to enter a discussion of RBF implementations of fuzzy logic;[5] the connection is obvious, and we forego this.

13.2.5. The Characteristic Strengths of RBF Classifiers

- Unlike most neural paradigms, RBF's radius-limited elements do not extend their interpolation arbitrarily far away from their control points (the exemplars). This gives them good false-positive rejection characteristics by avoiding uncontrolled regression.

- Because the elements do not communicate with each other, it is often possible to add/remove/combine goal classes without retraining existing elements.
- Because the elements have finite support, it is only necessary to fire those in the relevant region of feature space.
- RBF's are insensitive to the number of output classes. (We have successfully built and trained RBF's with over 300 output classes.)
- The decision parameters in RBF's have geometric significance.
- The components of the belief vector can be used to produce "confidence factors."
- The geometric/analytic nature of RBF's is exploitable using many conventional, mature mathematical tools.
- RBF's have been shown to have the theoretical power to handle arbitrary well-posed classification problems; non-linearly separable problems pose no special difficulty.
- Super-fast hardware implementations of RBF's are commercially available (c. 2 microseconds/classification, pipelined). The INTEL Ni1000 chip is the best example.
- RBF's can be designed to produce classifications of hierarchical "granularity." See the discussion of taxonomic decomposition below.

13.2.6. The Characteristic Weaknesses of RBF Classifiers

- Because RBF's model the data from many local approximations rather than from a few population parameters, they typical use more decision parameters than most other techniques (10,000 parameters is not unusual).
- RBF's are easy to "overtrain", that is, they can merely memorize idiosyncrasies of the training set rather than classification knowledge that will generalize.
- Because superposition is a "voting" strategy, RBF's can be sensitive to the presentation cardinalities in the training set.
- Management and use of the large number of RBF parameters can cause software implementations of RBF's to be slow.

- If every vector in an unambiguous training set is used as an exemplar for some basis function, the RBF will generally give a nearly perfect score on that training set; this makes RBF's hard to evaluate without using separate training and evaluation sets.

13.2.7. RBF Training

To train an RBF, we define an objective function, and perform non-linear optimization in parameter space. In general, this includes adjustment of both basis functions locations, and parameters. Geometrically, the RBF level-sets "float around and change shape" in an attempt to best cover clusters and portions of clusters present in the training set.

13.3. RBF Networks: Formal Definition

Mathematical construction of the Stage 1 RBF:

Let Feature space be $\mathbf{R}^{\mathbf{M}}$.

Let goal space G = {1, 2, ..., K}, so that points in $\mathbf{R}^{\mathbf{M}}$ fall into one of K classes.

Recall that "exemplars" are feature vectors which represent a particular class. Denote the ith of I exemplars for class *k* by:

$$\vec{F}_{ki} = f\left(f_{ki1},\ldots,f_{kiM}\right) \tag{13.1}$$

Define the basis function associated with $\vec{F}_{ki}$ by:

$$R_{ki}(\vec{x}) = 1 - Min\left(1, \sum_{m=1}^{M} P_{kim}(f_{kim} - x_m)^2\right) \tag{13.2}$$

where $\vec{x} = \left(x_1,\ldots,x_M\right) \in \mathbf{R}^{\mathbf{M}}$ and $\vec{P}_{ki} = \left(P_{ki1},\ldots,P_{kiM}\right)$ is a vector of (tunable) non-negative parameters. (Hence, for this implementation, parameter space is $\mathbf{R}^{\mathbf{M}}$).

R_{ki} establishes a hyper-elliptical (scalar) field of "belief" in k-membership around the exemplar $\vec{F}_{ki}$. R_{ki} has the following properties:

- the semi-major axes of the field are determined by the parameter vector $\vec{P}_{ki}$
- it is a monotone decreasing function of "elliptical distance" from $\vec{F}_{ki}$
- it attains its maximum of 1 precisely at $\vec{F}_{ki}$
- it is non-negative and has compact support
- it has continuous partials with respect to the parameters P_{kim} for all points having $R_{ki} > 0$.

$R_{ki}(\bar{x})$ is the contribution of exemplar $\bar{F}_{ki}$ to our belief that $\bar{x}$ is in class k.

Typically, there will be multiple exemplars for each class, so the "total belief" that a point $\bar{x}$ is in class k is an aggregation of the beliefs of the class k exemplars:

$$b_k(\bar{x}) = 1 - \prod_{i=1}^{I} \left(1 - R_{ki}(\bar{x})\right) \qquad (13.3)$$

This naturally gives rise to a vector field of beliefs $\mathbf{B}:\mathbf{R}^{\mathbf{M}} \to \mathbf{R}^{\mathbf{K}}$ defined by:

$$\bar{B}(\bar{x}) = \left(b_1(\bar{x}),\ldots,b_k(\bar{x})\right) \qquad (13.4)$$

$\bar{B}(\bar{x})$ can be interpreted as a joint-membership function, akin to a k-ary probability density.

$\bar{B}$ is the radial basis function constructed from the exemplars. It is trained by optimizing $\bar{P}_{ki}$.

To use $\bar{B}$ to classify points in feature space, select the index of the largest component of $\bar{B}(\bar{x})$. The b_k's can be used to build confidence factors.

For points far away from all exemplars ("uncontrolled" regions of feature space), $\bar{B}(\bar{x}) = \bar{0}$. The RBF refuses to make "wild guesses."

13.4. The Long-Term Load-Forecasting Problem

Long-term load forecasting is the prediction of load at an arbitrary future time. Since no "previous day" actual load data will be available to support such a forecast, long-term load prediction must be based exclusively on phenomenological factors (temporal and meteorological).

13.4.1. Data Collection

For this work, actual load data was provided at two feeders: feeder1 served just commercial users, and feeder2 served just residential users. Load was expressed in amps at 11 kV. Data were collected every 30 minutes (on the half-hour), 24 hours/day during the entire period from November 1, 1993 to October 31, 1994, a total of 17,520 load values for each feeder. All data were stamped with a date-time group.

Weather data was collected by a government meteorological station in the area. Weather data consisted of:

- Wet-bulb temperature (degrees Celsius)
- Dry-bulb temperature (degrees Celsius)
- Relative humidity (%)

- Wind direction (degrees of bearing)
- Wind speed (knots)
- Cloudiness factor (unitless, 1-10)

Data were collected every hour (on the hour), 24 hours/day during the entire period from November 1, 1993 to October 31, 1994, a total of 8,760 sets of readings. (Exception: cloudiness factor was collected only every 3 hours, at 0200, 0500, 0800, 1100, 1400, 1700, 2000, and 2300 hours).

NOTE: Commercial load forecasting and residential load forecasting were treated as completely separate problems. The commercial and residential data were not mixed or used jointly in any way for this study.

13.4.2. Selecting the Features

Because weather data was available only on the hour, the half-hourly load data was not used for this study. This left a common set of hourly load-weather data consisting of 8,760 data points for each of the commercial and residential sets.

Cloudiness factor was not selected, because it was available only for some hours.

For prototyping efficiency, it is desirable to keep the dimensionality of feature space as low as possible. The correlation coefficient of wind direction with load was very low, and the correlation coefficient of dry-bulb with wet-bulb temperature was very high (0.94). Therefore, wind direction and wet-bulb temperature were deemed irrelevant and redundant, respectively, and not selected.

This left a set of phenomenological features consisting of dry-bulb temperature, relative humidity, and wind speed.

Graphical display of the load data versus time showed consistent daily profiles. Three fundamental "day types" were observed: week-days (Monday-Friday); weekend-days (Saturday and Sunday); and holiday-days (e.g., Christmas Day). "Day type" was selected as a feature.

Month and hour-of-day were seen to be correlated with load, and were selected as features.

This gives a set of temporal features consisting of month, day-of-week, and day type.

Thus, the selection process yielded a set of six temporal-meteorological features: Month, day type, hour-of-day, dry-bulb temperature, relative humidity, and wind speed.

NOTE: We were told by the providers of the load data that other useful features existed, but were proprietary. These features are anticipated to be available for follow-on work.

13.4.3. Coding the Feature Vectors

How shall features be represented within the feature vector? A naive representation of time by hour number would tell the RBF that 11 p.m., which has representation "23", is very far in feature space from midnight, which has representation "0." Similarly, December ("12") would be presented to the RBF as very far in feature space from January ("1").

Also, relative humidity represented in percentage points attains much higher numeric values, and has greater dynamic range than any other feature, for example. And, what should be the representation of day type?

A partial solution to the representation problem is offered by principle component analysis (PCA). This handles range and centering variations, but destroys the semantic identify of the features, which is needed for experimental work. (Note: The Karhunen-Loeve transform is a standard PCA technique used in classification work for feature set conditioning.)

For this study, month and hour-of-day were coded by their corresponding average temperature. That is, the month January was represented in the feature vector as 20.4, the average temperature during January. Similarly, for example, 8 a.m. was represented as 13.8, the average temperature (over the whole year) at that time. (It would be preferable to code these variables by average load, the variable to be predicted, but we wanted to avoid overuse of the load data.)

The humidity data were linearly rescaled to be in the range 0 - 20 (and so roughly commensurable with the temperature data.) Wind speed data were not coded.

Day type was coded to show that holidays and weekends had similar average load levels, both of which were very different, and less than, weekday levels: holiday = 1, weekend = 4, weekday = 12.

13.5. The Load-Forecasting Problem as a Classification Problem

Since load is a continuous random variable, an RBF classifier might appear ill-suited to load prediction. We posed the problem in terms of classification to exploit the RBF's controlled regression, and guarantee the existence of a development path to an ultra-high-throughput hardware implementation.

13.5.1. Day Profiles and Quantized Correction Factors

For each of the seven days of the week, a load profile was computed. This profile was the entire year's arithmetic average of the 24 hourly loads for that day of the week. for example, the Monday profile consists of 24 loads: the hour-0 load is the average of the entire year's Monday at 1 a.m. loads, etc. The Monday profile, then, is the waveform of hourly loads for the "average Monday." A profile was also prepared for the average holiday, giving a total of 8 day-of-week load profiles.

Because the day profiles are only gross averages, and do not take phenomenological features into account, they will be weak predictors. For any particular date and time, the actual measured load will usually be different from the profile load for that day of the week. The ratio:

$$F = (\text{actual load}) \,/\, (\text{profile load}) \qquad (13.5)$$

gives a correction factor for that date and time. If we could predict, from temporal and meteorological features, what correction factor to apply to the profile load, the profile could be corrected to a predicted load.

This is the approach taken under this study. In this way, by quantizing the range of multipliers observed (0.5 - 1.5, roughly), the load prediction problem is recast. It becomes the problem of selecting the correct one of (finitely many) quantization bins for the correction factor: we have a classification problem.

The approach may be stated:

- The interval from 0.5 to 1.5 is divided into a finite number of bins. The midpoint (for example) of each bin is its reconstruction value, F.
- For each of the feature vectors in the training set, we compute what the correction value F from profile load to actual load is. The bin number containing this multiplier F becomes the desired output of the RBF for this feature vector. This output is an integer.
- The RBF is trained to produce the desired bin number as its output.

To use the RBF as a load predictor:

- Input a feature vector of temporal and meteorological features. Using these feature as input, the RBF returns a bin number, which corresponds to a known correction factor, F.
- Multiply the profile value for the desired hour/day-of-week by the factor F to obtain the load prediction.

The study RBF is seen to be a machine which computes single-point corrections to a template based upon phenomenological data. Notice that the RBF must be run for each prediction desired, so prediction of an entire day's data requires 24 runs.

13.5.2. The Training Set

Examination of the 365 days of available feature vector revealed 14 days with corrupted data (typically, drop-outs resulting from sensors going off-line). These days were not considered during exemplar selection, leaving 351 days of data, having a total of 24 * 351 = 8,424 feature vectors.

13.5.3. Training the Stage 1 RBF

A recursive "taxonomic" decomposition of the feature space was performed.

To begin the decomposition, a single exemplar was computed for each class. This synthesized exemplar was the unweighted mean of the feature vectors of that class. For each of these COG's ("centers of gravity") semi-major axes were computed to be the standard deviations in each dimension. Hence, the initial untrained RBF was essentially a k-means classifier. By a nearest-neighbor rule, this decomposes feature space into regions by proximity to exemplars.

Since, in general, classes will not manifest as disjoint convex clusters in feature space, the initial decomposition will have ambiguous (i.e., multi-class) regions. We optimize, adjusting the RBF exemplars (COG's) and semi-major axes (parameters) by maximizing an objective function. This optimization is performed using a gradient-assisted generate-and-test algorithm in parameter space.

When optimization is complete, feature space has been decomposed into subregions which are, to the extent possible, homogeneous by class (as determined with respect to the training set). This decomposition procedure is then applied to each of these subregions. A hierarchical taxonomic decomposition of feature space results. This process is continued until the regions at the bottom of the tree consist of disjoint convex clusters, or can be handled by an individual MLP tied to that terminal-sub-region.

The taxonomic decomposition is similar to a quadtree decomposition, except that the space partitioning is driven by the class-distribution of exemplars. The stage 1 RBF classifies feature vectors by determining into which terminal region they are placed in accordance with the hierarchy.

13.5.4. Determining When the Stage 1 RBF has Improved

The objective function has two parts, called scores. Score A is the percent of feature vectors in the training set correctly classified by the stage 1 RBF. Score B is the "disambiguity." For training, the RBF is considered to have improved when:

- score A increases, without respect to the change in score B
- Score A is unchanged, and score B increases

It remains to describe the disambiguity. In general, cluster centers and sizes have been well-chosen when intra-cluster distances are small, inter-cluster distances are large, and clusters are widely separated.

Let $S_1(i)$ be the sum of the distances of all class i feature vectors from the class i exemplar (the "intra-score"). Let $S_2(i)$ be the sum of the distances from the class i exemplar to all feature vectors not in class i (the "inter-score"). Let S_3 be the sum of the distances of all exemplars each other.

Let X_1 be the sum of the $S_1(i)$, and let X_2 be the sum of the $S_2(i)$.

Good clustering will have a smaller X_1 value, and larger X_2 and S_3 values. To capture this in a single value, we set:

$$\text{Disambiguity} = \text{Score B} = X_1 / (1 + X_2 * S_3) \qquad (13.6)$$

13.5.5. Smoothing as a Post-Process

The study prototype does not take into account the fact there is a "behavior lag" inherent in utility loads: consumers do not respond to weather conditions continuously and in real-time; rather, they tend to set their consumption based upon recent experience and perceived trends. It was found that this could be partially compensated for by spatial smoothing of the predicted load waveforms with a rastered average filter. A 3-hour wide, centered-output window with uniform weights was used.

13.6. Results

Evaluation testing was against the whole 365 days of feature vectors (includes "bad" days), and so constituted a test which was over 80% "blind", and included nearly 4% "real-world" anomalous input.

The current customary error measurement for load prediction in the literature seems to be "RMS % of peak load" (RMS%pl). That is, an RMS error is computed over the entire prediction period (usually 24 hours), divided by the period's peak load, and multiplied by 100%.

Short-term load predictors typically use previous-day load data, and perform at a nominal 2% error (RMS%pl).

13.6.1. Residential Feeder

The RBF was trained on the residential feeder data. Using six output quantization bins, the study RBF reconstructed the entire year's residential loads from the corresponding meteorological data. It performed at 9.1% error (RMS%pl). The error computation period was the whole year.

13.6.2. Commercial Feeder

The same RBF was retrained on the commercial feeder data. Using six output quantization bins, the study RBF reconstructed the entire year's commercial loads from the corresponding meteorological data. It performed at 6.9% error (RMS%pl). The error computation period was the whole year.

Note: Of the 1,685 feature vectors that were in the training set, the RBF returned the correct quantization bin 1,682 times, an accuracy of 99.8%.

Experiments were conducted at various quantization levels, using up to 120 bins. Results did not vary much with the number of quantization bins, though ambiguities in the training set (i.e., same weather data, different desired load) did show up when using more bins.

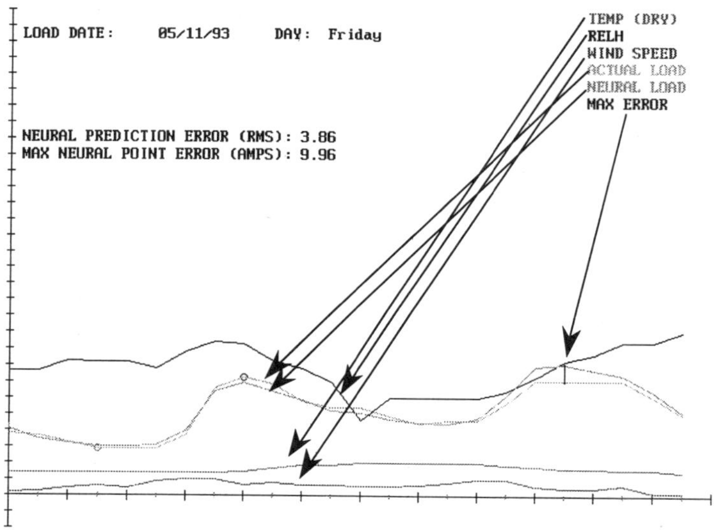

Figure 13.2. An RBF Prediction for a Residential Day.

13.6.3. Implementation/Performance

The RBF software for this study was developed under previous IR&D. The analysis and development for this study was conducted under a rapid prototyping methodology in 30 man-days. It has a simple semi-graphical color MMI, and consists of about 1,200 lines of high-order compiled code running on a 486 50 MHz PC clone. Several analysis routines and support utilities were developed as part of this effort.

The prototype produced under this study requires about 2 hours to train, and performs a single-point load prediction in about 300 milliseconds.

Note that the effectiveness of any predictive model is affected by the user's ability to predict the input parameters. For load prediction, these parameters include weather data.

13.7. Future Work

The results obtained under this study exceeded expectations in terms of predictive power and throughput. Based upon these results, commercial funding for additional work is now being negotiated.

There are 11 enhancements proposed for future work:

- Use more than 1,685 training vectors, from multiple years, and select these intelligently.
- Use finer stratification (e.g., monthly) for generating day templates.
- Do not include corrupt data in the test suite.
- Use some load data in preparing/coding feature vectors.
- Apply better conditioning (e.g., PCA) to feature sets.
- Use proprietary features.
- Optimize code for throughput.
- Apply/evaluate other RBF models.
- Optimize quantization of reconstruction values (e.g., Max quantization).
- Use incremental confidence factors to evaluate output.
- Account for behavior lag.

13.8. Biography

Monte F. Hancock, Jr., MS is Chief Scientist and Director of Research and Development at CSI, and also serves on the Adjunct Facility of Rollins College, in the Departments of Mathematics and Computer Science. He is listed in the current edition of "Who's Who in the South and Southwest."

Computer Science Innovations, Inc. was founded in 1983 in Palm Bay, Florida and is currently active in a wide variety of markets. From a beginning based on the design and development of custom, state-of-the-art Information Management Systems for the Command, Control, Communications and Intelligence (C^3I)

marketplace, CSI now participates in both DoD and commercial markets. CSI's main business is solving our customers hardest problems using innovative solutions and the latest in technology.

CSI is headquartered in Melbourne, Florida and has branch offices in the Baltimore-Washington area and Central America.

Tel: (407) 676-2923 Fax: (407) 676-2355

13.9. References

Hecht-Nielsen's book is undoubtedly the best general reference available on neural networks. The author knows of no definitive general reference on radial basis functions. The RBF paradigm is a little over 10 years old.

1. R. Hecht-Nielsen, *Neurocomputing* (Addison-Wesley, 1990), p. 7.
2. B. Kosko, *Neural Networks for Signal Processing* (Prentice Hall, 1992).
3. J. Dugundji, *Topology* (Allyn and Bacon, 1973), pp. 169-171.
4. E. Rich and K. Knight, *Artificial Intelligence* (McGraw-Hill, 1991), pp. 492-500.
5. B. Kosko, *Neural Networks and Fuzzy Systems* (Prentice Hall, 1992).

13.10. Bibliography

D. W. Bunn, "Short-Term Load Forecasting: A Review of Procedures in the Electric Supply Industry," *J. Opl. Res. Soc.* **33** (1982) 533-545.

S.T. Chen, "Weather Sensitive Short-Term Load Forecasting Using Neural Networks," *IEEE Transactions of Power Systems* (August 1992).

Engle and Goodrich, *Forecasting Electricity Sales Over the Short-Term: A comparison of New Methodologies* (Electric Power Research Institute, Palo Alto, CA, 1986), Report No. EM-4772.

G. Gross and F. D. Galiana, "Short Term Load Forecasting," *Proc. IEEE* **75** (1987) 1558-1973.

I. Moghram and S. Rahman, "Analysis and Evaluation of Five Short-Term Load Forecasting Techniques," *IEEE Transactions on Power Systems* **4** (1989) 1484-1490.

14. AN APPROACH TO DISTRIBUTION SHORT-TERM LOAD FORECASTING

REX (TRAV) C. STRATTON AND KRISTA L. GAUSTAD
Pacific Northwest National Laboratory†*, P.O. Box 999, {MS K7-28 and MS K5-20}*
Richland, Washington 99352, USA
E-mail: rc_stratton@pnl.gov, kl_gaustad@pnl.gov

ABSTRACT

This paper reports on the developments and findings of the Distribution Short-Term Load Forecaster (DSTLF) research activity. The objective of this research is to develop a distribution short-term load forecasting technology consisting of a forecasting method, development methodology, theories necessary to support required technical components, and the hardware and software tools required to perform the forecast. The DSTLF consists of four major components: monitored endpoint load forecaster (MELF), nonmonitored endpoint load forecaster (NELF), topological integration forecaster (TIF), and a dynamic tuner. These components interact to provide short-term forecasts at various points in the distribution system, e.g., feeder, line section, and endpoint. This paper discusses the DSTLF methodology and MELF component. MELF, based on artificial neural network technology, predicts distribution endpoint loads for an hour, a day, and a week in advance. Predictions are developed using time, calendar, historical load, and weather data. The overall DSTLF architecture and a prototype MELF module for retail endpoints have been developed. Future work will be focused on refining and extending MELF and developing NELF and TIF capabilities.

14.1. Introduction

14.1.1. New Requirements on the Distribution System

A number of recent developments have resulted in several challenges to the electric power industry. Among the most influential factors are increased power flow on existing systems, the expansion of distributed automation and demand-side management (DA/DSM) activities, deregulation, and the installation of generation at the distribution level. Each of these factors has the potential to significantly alter the design, operation, and maintenance requirements of the distribution systems. A proposed method of alleviating anticipated technical difficulties is to automate the distri-

†This work was supported by the Laboratory Directed Research and Development Program at Pacific Northwest National Laboratory (PNNL). PNNL is a multiprogram national laboratory operated by Battelle Memorial Institute for the U.S. Department of Energy under Contract DE-AC06-76RLO 1830.

bution system. Appropriate automation can increase operating flexibility and speed, defer requirements for costly transmission and generation improvements (by increasing utilization of available resources), and improve power reliability and quality.

The ability to make accurate short-term load predictions on distribution feeders will be vital to optimizing distribution system operations and maintenance. In particular, the ability to plan for system power requirements an hour to a week ahead is critical to a number of real-time control requirements (e.g., economic generating capacity scheduling, fuel purchase scheduling, security analysis, transaction evaluation, power flow and switching cycle optimization, and distribution reconfiguration). Such capability is necessary to ensure power system stability under high load demands, to perform DSM load management activities, to optimally configure the system for current/near-term conditions, and to economically optimize system operation with respect to power flow/generation.

14.1.2. Objective

The Pacific Northwest National Laboratory (PNNL) is currently conducting a multiyear research project to develop a core technology for building short-term load forecasters. These forecasters will accurately predict load requirements at the distribution level of the power system. The project supports a recently initiated research activity focused toward appropriately applying intelligent information technology (IIT) to the electric power industry transmission and distribution sector.

The Distribution Short-Term Load Forecaster (DSTLF) consists of four major components: monitored endpoint load forecaster (MELF), nonmonitored endpoint load forecaster (NELF), topological integration forecaster (TIF), and dynamic tuner. These components interact to provide short-term forecasts at various points in the distribution system, i.e., substation, feeder, line section, and endpoint. Loads will be predicted for a period of time between one hour and one week into the future.

Because load characteristics in a power system change over time as a function of economics, technology, conservation, and population demographics, the DSTLFs must be able to monitor their own performance and self-tune, should that performance fall below a specified threshold. This self-tuning capability will also increase flexibility during the installation process. It is also anticipated that as monitoring capabilities for distribution systems are upgraded, an insufficient amount of historical data will be available to pretrain DSTLFs for site-specific load characteristics. Self-tuning forecasters trained for a site with load characteristics similar to those for the desired location can be installed and allowed to improve their accuracy over time as experience is gained.

This paper reports on the first year of the DSTLF research efforts. The general DSTLF methodology and initial MELF development efforts will be discussed in detail.

14.2. Load Forecasting Background

Load forecasting is the process of predicting the electrical load on a power system for some period of time in the future. The forecasts are typically based on knowledge of system composition, historical load behavior, and weather. Load forecasts are made for both long and short periods of time. Short-term forecasts are used in near-term decision processes and to maintain the day-to-day operation of the power system. Applications requiring short-term load forecasting (STLF) capabilities include power system control, scheduling, and security.

14.2.1. Short-Term Load Forecasting (STLF) Methods

At the transmission level, STLF has traditionally been performed using either a time-series or regression method. Time-series methods treat the load pattern as a time-series signal with known periodicities and predict the future load by using various time-series analysis techniques such as Kalman filtering, autoregressive-moving average (ARMA), and Box-Jenkins.[1] In contrast, regression methods use a linear or piecewise-linear function to represent the functional relationship between pertinent variables (e.g., weather, customer usage) and system load. Load is predicted by inserting the weather information into the predetermined functional relationship.[1]

Both time-series and regression methods involve complex modeling techniques and have heavy computational requirements resulting in long computational times and a tendency to experience numerical instabilities. These inherent drawbacks have stimulated development of forecasters based on artificial intelligence (AI). Both expert systems and artificial neural networks have been applied to the load forecasting problem.

Expert systems use the knowledge of a human expert to develop rules for forecasting. Artificial neural networks (ANNs) do not rely on human experience but attempt to draw a link between sets of input data and observed output. Although the accuracy of load predictions made by expert systems and ANNs is relatively the same, the difficulty in acquiring and transforming the knowledge of an expert to a set of rules makes ANN technology slightly more attractive for STLF applications.

ANN technology has proven to be a viable option to statistical techniques such as regression analysis, time-series prediction, and classification. The advantages of ANNs in statistical applications include robustness to probability distribution assumptions, their ability to classify in the presence of nonlinear separation surfaces, and their ability to perform reasonably well with incomplete data.[2] ANN technologies have been selected to form the basis of PNNL's distribution system MELF development. An overview of ANN technology can be found in References 1-4.

Although a significant amount of research has been conducted in the past five years with respect to the use of ANNs in short-term load forecasting, much of the development has been focused on predicting load at the transmission level. Inherent differences in the makeup and operating characteristics of distribution and transmission systems will prevent the direct transfer of traditional transmission-level statistical techniques and AI STLFing technologies to the distribution level. The development of an efficient method of predicting loads at the distribution level will depend on an understanding of distribution system characteristics that complicate the short-term load forecasting process.

14.2.2. Distribution Short-Term Load Forecasting Issues

The unique features of the distribution system could impede DSTLF development efforts. Distribution system characteristics that will complicate the development of DSTLFs include the lack of historical data, dynamic changes in distribution system configuration, sparse sensing, and the increased randomness associated with single endpoint load shapes.

Independent of the forecasting technique used, the fundamental requirement for successful STLF is access to historical hourly data of the proper quality and quantity. Presently, distribution systems can be characterized as data- poor with respect to both data quality and quantity. ANN (and other) STLF techniques are based on knowledge of the load shape provided by historical hourly load and weather data. The ANN training data needs to be as accurate and complete as possible.

An additional difficulty associated with predicting distribution system loads is the dynamic nature of the distribution system physical configuration. To maximize the reliability of the system and maintain services to the customer, the physical layout of the distribution system is reconfigured. This reconfiguration is performed manually or automatically, often with little warning. The number and nature of endpoints on a feeder can change, thus changing characteristics of the loadshape. A DSTLF must be able to adapt, in real time, to any topological changes in the distribution network. The concept of the TIF component of the DSTLF and the self-tuning capability were developed to address the issues associated with the dynamic nature of the distribution system.

Finally, the very nature of the load at the distribution level complicates development of a DSTLF. The number of individual loads represented by a distribution feeder is much smaller than the number of individual loads that comprise a transmission line. Load forecasts made at transmission levels benefit from the larger number of endpoints based on the law of large numbers. The law of large numbers dictates that the impact of unusual characteristics and anomalies tends to be minimized when a large number of data points is included in the analysis, thus increasing the accuracy of predictions. In addition to the statistical difficulty associated with analysis of a large number of endpoints, the load shape of a single endpoint will have larger relative changes in load and will be significantly affected by unusual events or sudden changes.

Current developments in the power industry are bringing the need for automated short-term prediction capabilities to the forefront of distribution system improvement efforts. The unique features of the distribution system will complicate STLF development efforts. The success of the DSTLF core technology will depend, in part, on how well the DSTLF methodology and its associated elements (MELF, NELF, TIF, and dynamic tuner) address the limited monitoring, dynamic state, and variability of load.

14.3. DSTLF Methodology

PNNL has defined a DSTLF methodology that addresses the changing utility industry's needs and the unique distribution system forecasting environment. The methodology is designed to facilitate the development of a core forecasting technology that is pervasive across all distribution systems and independent of a utility's monitoring scheme, physical layout, and endpoint characteristics. The capabilities required to develop the methodology elements include a load forecasting method, load shape group/type identification, endpoint load aggregation, and dynamic self-tuning.

14.3.1. Methodology Basis

Methods for forecasting load at any level of a power system are constrained by the type and amount of data gathered from the network. Because of the lack of data at the distribution level, the forecasting method is based on limited monitoring of endpoint loads but will accommodate and, in fact, be more accurate with increased monitoring. In a limited monitoring environment, a certain percentage of endpoints is continuously monitored. Loads for the monitored endpoints are directly forecasted from the gathered data. Loads for nonmonitored endpoints are estimated based on analysis of load characteristics of similar monitored endpoints using a group/type characterization scheme that matches endpoints with similar properties and load shapes.

Because current distribution systems are poorly monitored, the development of a robust group/type characterization scheme is essential for forecasting load at the distribution level. At this time, a proven group/type method that characterizes load shapes of endpoints based on the load behavior of other endpoints in the same group/type does not exist. PNNL's research will answer a fundamental question: can grouping schemes be developed that cluster endpoints with similar load shapes to a degree that meets the industry's performance requirements?

Once both monitored and nonmonitored endpoint loads have been predicted, line, feeder, and substation loads can be estimated by employing an aggregation method that sums endpoint loads located on the respective line sections and feeders. Line losses should be accounted for in the summing process.

The self-tuning feature allows the DSTLF to adapt to the changing network environment. Self-tuning is a gradual process. Following a change in the physical configuration or in the nature of the loads on the system, the accuracy of the DSTLF will decrease and then improve as tuning progresses. Because of the initial decrease in performance, the DSTLF system should be able to anticipate potential configuration scenarios. An automated configuration management system is necessary to support DSTLF activities and provide the information necessary to pretune the DSTLF based on expected physical layouts.

The DSTLF development process and core components were defined to address the issues associated with the limited monitoring environment as well as the group/type, aggregation, and dynamic self-tuning requirements that form the basis of DSTLF methodology.

14.3.2 Methodology Description

The DSTLF methodology is described in terms of the data requirements, the processes the data undergoes, and the DSTLF components that perform the data processing activities. Layered data process modules are used to illustrate the interactions between the data and core component processing elements, the interactions between the various core component processing elements themselves, and the process flow required to obtain the desired forecasted load.

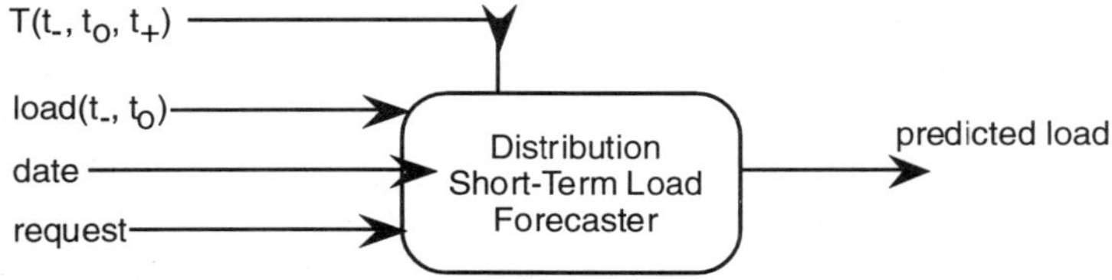

Figure 14.1. Distribution Short-Term Load Forecaster (DSTLF).

The input data required by the DSTLF, shown in Figure 14.1, is dependent on the forecasting technology, the group/type theory, and the aggregation and self-tuning methods. Input data typically consists of historical load, historical temperature, current load, current temperature, and the forecast request.

The approach for predicting a load is to estimate the load of monitored endpoints, use the resulting forecasts, in conjunction with group/typing schemes, to predict the loads of nonmonitored endpoints, and aggregate the individual endpoint forecasts, as necessary, to estimate line and feeder loads. These processes are performed by the monitored endpoint load forecaster (MELF), nonmonitored endpoint load forecaster (NELF), and topological integration forecaster (TIF), respectively.

The MELF consists of a forecasting element based on ANN technology trained from historical data to predict the load of an endpoint (or a specific location on a distribution system). The MELF ANN design and development processes have been conducted with the goal of eventually automating the process. The MELF's ANN has two operational modes: a learning mode, during which the weights associated with the interconnecting nodes are optimized, and a forecasting mode, during which requested load forecasts are made. The learning mode is invoked prior to integration with the other DSTLF elements and as needed by the dynamic tuner element.

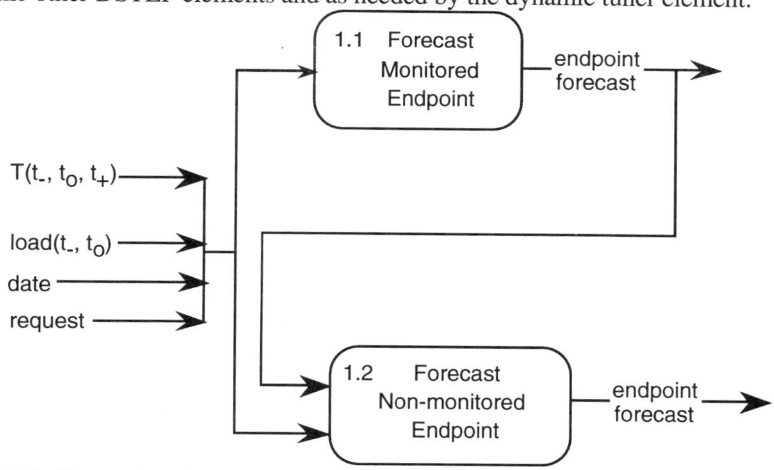

Figure 14.2. Nonmonitored Endpoint Load Forecaster (NELF).

The MELF-predicted forecasts are used either directly (if the load is for a monitored endpoint) or as input to the NELF. The relationship between the MELF and NELF is shown in Figure 14.2. The NELF consists of a group/typing scheme and one or more transform algorithms. A NELF operates by using a group/typing scheme to identify MELF(s) with similar behavior characteristics. The forecast, generated by the MELF, and the nonmonitored endpoint historical and real-time data are analyzed by the NELF to identify the transform algorithm needed to forecast the desired endpoint's load. If the group/type analysis determines that an endpoint belongs to multiple groups, additional transform algorithms will be required to individually assess the contribution of each group to the endpoint's total load.

If the requested load is for a point in the distribution system that consists of multiple endpoint loads (e.g., a line section, feeder, or substation) and the point is not directly monitored, the TIF estimates the load by summing the endpoints associated with the location. The TIF uses a topological model to identify the endpoints associated with a specific location in the distribution system. The model describes the system in terms of endpoints, cable, and switches, fuses, and other components that can change the configuration. Predictions can be made for both the current and potential physical configurations. The TIF also address issues associated with the aggregation process such as line losses. Figure 14.3 shows the relationship between endpoint, line, and feeder forecasts.

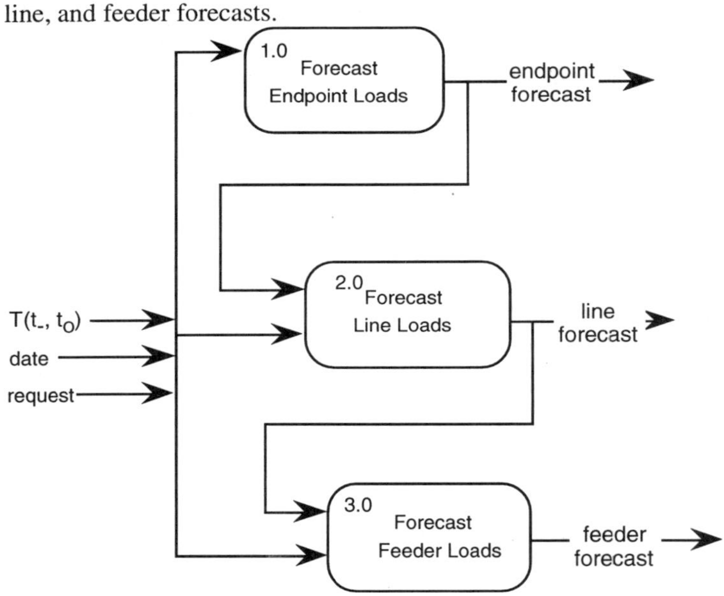

Figure 14.3. Topological Integration Forecaster (TIF).

Input data is used directly by the line and feeder forecasters if the line or feeder is directly monitored. Endpoint forecasts are used as input data if they are not directly monitored.

14.3.3. AI Technology Requirements

A number of AI technologies will be used to develop the DSTLF capability. Previous research experience in building intelligent software systems has indicated a benefit associated with integrating diverse AI paradigms. The DSTLF will employ ANNs, fuzzy logic, and model-based reasoning.

Because the nonlinearity and statistical nature of endpoint load profiles are well suited to prediction by neural networks, ANNs form the basis of the load forecasting technology used by the MELF.

Fuzzy logic is well suited for forecasting the loads of nonmonitored endpoints because of the subjective group/type schemes and issues associated with membership. The group/type theory will provide a crisp definition of ideal group types. However, actual endpoints will most likely not be ideal and may share properties with more than one group/type. Fuzzy logic is an appropriate technology for capturing inexactness in grouping processes and provides logical inferencing and computation capabilities.

The TIF will use model-based reasoning techniques to identify the preferred configuration for a given set of operating conditions and requirements. The TIF will examine models representing the current and potential physical layouts of the distribution system and power system analysis models representing the current and potential operating conditions of the distribution system.

Model-based reasoning technology will be used also in developing a dynamic self-tuner. The basic approach will be to combine a performance reasoner with the ANN learning algorithm. The performance reasoner will detect the need for adjusting the weights of the MELF and, based on this detection, will implement the learning algorithm. Subsequent to implementing the new weights, the performance will be compared to the existing forecaster's accuracy. Based on the results of the comparison, the revised weights will be substituted for the current weights, or further evaluation and training will take place.

14.4. Summary

Accomplishments during the first year of the DSTLF development include the establishment of a DSTLF concept, partial development of an overall DSTLF methodology, and completion of proof-of-concept prototype MELFs.

The first year of DSTLF research has provided sufficient proof of concept to continue development efforts. In addition, it has produced a framework to guide future development efforts. Ongoing efforts that will be continued include general MELF prototype development and completion of the DSTLF methodology. Remaining elements of the DSTLF that will also be pursued include the group/type theory, NELF, topological integrator, and self-tuning capability. Because of the distribution industry's nearly universal limited endpoint monitoring environment, near-term activities will focus on development of a group/type theory.

14.5. Biographies

Trav Stratton received his B.S. in Physics and M.S. in nuclear engineering from Texas A&M University in 1971 and 1975, respectively. He joined Pacific Northwest National Laboratory in 1987. His interests include artificial intelligence research and application development for reasoning about physical systems with a focus on the diagnosis of components.

Krista Gaustad received her B.E.E. and M.S. in electrical engineering from Auburn University in 1989 and 1991 respectively. She joined Pacific Northwest National Laboratory in 1991. Her interests include the application of intelligent information technologies to the electric power industry.

14.6. Acknowledgment

The concept of utilizing group/typing theories to estimate the load at nonmonitored endpoints was developed by Dr. Keyhani of Ohio State University. The proposed D-STLF methodology is based in part on a methodology conceived by Pacific Gas & Electric staff in conjunction with Dr. Keyhani.

14.7. References

1. D.C. Park, M.A. El-Sharkawi, R.J. Marks II, L.I. Atlas and M.J. Damborg, "Electric Load Forecasting Using an Artificial Neural Network," *IEEE Transactions on Power Systems* **6(2)** (May 1991).
2. Alex Papalexopoulos, D. Shangyou Hao and Tie-Mao Peng, "Application of Neural Network Technology to Short-Term System Load Forecasting," Presented at the *Athens Power Technology Conference* (Athens, Greece, Sept. 1993).
3. Alireza Khotanzad, Rey-Chue Hwang and Dominic Maratukulam, "Hourly Load Forecasting by Neural Networks," presented at a session entitled "Application of Neural Networks to Short-Term Load Forecasting" held at *IEEE PES Winter Meeting* (Columbus, Ohio, Feb. 1993).
4. K.Y. Lee, Y.T. Cha and J.H. Park, "Short-Term Load Forecasting Using An Artificial Neural Network," *Transactions on Power Systems* **7(1)** (Feb. 1992).

15. TWIN SIGNAL SENSING: APPLICATION TO SHORTED WINDING MONITORING, DETECTION AND LOCALIZATION

ROBERT J. STREIFEL, ROBERT J. MARKS II, M.A. EL-SHARKAWI, AND I. KERSZENBAUM

Department of Electrical Engineering, University of Washington, Box 352500
Seattle, Washington 98195-2500, USA

E-mail: streifel@ee.washington.edu, marks@ee.washington.edu, elsharkawi@ee.washington.edu

ABSTRACT

Using twin signal sensing we propose a method to monitor, detect and localize shorts in power system devices with windings: including rotors, transformers and motors. There has, to date, been no effective way to do so. The most obvious approach, time domain reflectometry, fails due to the reactive coupling of the windings.

Twin signal signature sensing of shorts results from identical signals being simultaneously injected in both sides of the windings. The reflected signals are measured and the difference amplified to produce the signature signal. The signature signal characterizes the current state of the windings. When winding shorts are present, the electrical characteristics of the device will be different and thus the signature signal will also change. The changes in the signature signal can be monitored to detect shorted windings.

While a device is in operation, the signature signals can be monitored and the development of winding shorts can be diagnosed through the process of novelty detection. After a device is cleaned or otherwise known to be functioning correctly (no winding shorts), signature signals can be collected which represent the healthy device. If a sufficient number of signals can be collected, the signal space representing healthy windings can be characterized. A detection surface can be placed around the healthy signature signals to provide a partition of the signal space into two regions: healthy and faulty. Any signature signal which is not within the healthy signature partition will indicate a faulted device.

Early tests of this technique have shown promise. Using an autotransformer, signatures were recorded and a spherical surface constructed around the healthy signals. Shorts were then introduced in the windings of the transformer and the signatures recorded. The novelty detector correctly identified all signatures, healthy and faulted. Since the transformer was not in operation and represents a rather easy detection problem, signature signals for two large turbogenerators were collected for further analysis. The signature signals for a rotating machine will differ significantly from the signatures of a dismantled rotor due to the effects of the brushes and the additional reflection path available through the excitation source. Rotation of a device will also affect the signature signals. Therefore, signature signals collected while the rotor is dismantled cannot be used for detecting shorted windings in an operational rotor.

Dismantling and reassembling a large turbogenerator is extremely expensive and time consuming. The introduction of artificial shorts in the windings is thus not possible. Due to the inability to induce shorts into these large machines while in operation, tests have been inconclusive so far. Work is now underway to allow testing of the novelty detection technique on a small laboratory machine.

When a device is out of service and shorts can be induced, signature signals can be collected. Windings which have been previously fingerprinted can be subjected to tests to localize the shorts. The standard layered perceptron neural network appears ideal to make these decisions. When the device is out of service, shorts can be introduced at a variety of locations, and a neural network trained to recognize the signature signals and identify the shorted turn location.

The signature signals are sampled and represent high dimensional vectors. Since these high dimensional vectors prohibit rapid learning by the neural network, features are extracted prior to training. The features are extracted by computing the area under the signature signal within specified time intervals. The signature signal is divided into 13 regions, more closely spaced near the origin, to provide adequate features.

The neural network performs pattern classification by identifying the shorted turn number given the signature signal. In normal pattern classification applications, a neuron is required for each output class. In the localization of shorted windings, a neuron would be required for each winding. Since the number of windings can be rather large and a large number of output neurons can cause slow learning, the concept of a fuzzified neuron is used.[1] The output of each neuron is trained to produce a standard triangular membership function. Two membership functions overlap the same space and the neuron outputs sum to one. This technique reduces the dimensionality of the network output by allowing interpolation and provides a filtered output from the network. See Reference 1 for details.

The rotor of a 60 MVA turbogenerator was used to test these ideas. The rotor had 14 coils with 17 turns in each coil. After training of the neural network, the network correctly identified all coils with shorted turns and predicted the shorted turn number to within 7 turns.

Preliminary work, performed on both downed and rotating loaded rotors, has been quite promising in demonstrating the effectiveness of the twin signal signature sensing approach to winding short evolution monitoring.

15.1. Reference

1. M.A. El-Sharkawi, R.J. Marks II, S. Oh, S.J. Huang, I. Kerszenbaum and A. Rodriquez, "Localization of Winding Shorts Using Fuzzified Neural Networks," in *Proceedings of the 1994 IEEE PES Winter Meeting*, (IEEE, New York, 1994).

16. DESIGN OF A HYBRID WIND POWER STORAGE AND GENERATION SYSTEM FOR A REMOTE COMMUNITY

SATINDERPAUL S. DEVGAN AND DUSTY R. WALKER, JR.
Department of Electrical and Computer Engineering, Tennessee State University
Nashville, Tennessee 37209-1561, USA
E-mail: sdevgan@harpo.tnstate.edu

ABSTRACT

There are thousands of small communities in various parts of the world, even in developed countries, that are too far away to be economically connected to an electric supply system. Clean water is essential for health and well being and electric energy is essential for economic development of the community. This paper describes the design of a "hybrid" Wind/Diesel power generation and storage system, and the electric power distribution system for a small rural community of 50 persons and live stock. The most cost effective and reliable system designed to satisfy reasonable growth over the next twenty-five years consists of three 10 kW wind turbines, a 30 kWh storage battery and a 17.5 kW backup diesel generator. This paper also describe efforts to train a neural network to predict wind power over the next time interval and few more time intervals. This is very essential for significant penetration of wind power systems.

16.1. Introduction

Availability of clean water and reliable electric energy supply are very important for the health and economic well being of a community. There are over two million homes in the United States that have no electric power supply and are too far away from a power grid to be economically connected to it. Furthermore with the world population projected to reach about 8.1 billion in 2020,[1,4] most people will probably find accommodations that may be too far away from any power station. They may find alternate renewable energy sources more economical than a connection to an utility line.

About 78% of the energy produced today is from fossil fuels. These fuels produce CO_2, and other gases that lead to the greenhouse effect or global warming.[1] Also, coal burning produces SO_2 which leads to acid rain effect. The Clean Air Act Amendments[2] of 1990 and the recently passed Energy Policy Act of 1992 along with state regulatory commissions are encouraging electric utilities to use cost-effective renewable energy systems as part of their generation mix. The US "Climatic Change Action Plan" calls for greenhouse effect related emissions to not exceed the

†This work was supported in part by the U.S. Department of Energy's National Renewable Energy Laboratory (NREL) under sub-contract Number XAH-3-13203-01.

1990 levels by year 2000.[3,4] If the present trend in energy production continues, the CO_2 emission will increase from the current level of 358 parts per million to 600 parts per million in 2100[3,5] which may lead to serious health problems for many people.

In the past remote communities and towns that needed electricity, relied upon diesel/generator sets as sources of electric power. As our society is getting technically advanced, there is an ever increasing need for more reliable, environmentally safe, and cost effective means of producing and distributing electric energy. With a capacity of providing up to ten percent (10%) of America's energy needs, wind turbines are available to generate electricity over ninety-seven percent (97%) of the time, and can operate over 6,000 hours per year.[6] Already next generation wind turbines are bidding to produce electricity for four (4) cents per kilo-watt-hour by 1995. The advances in wind turbine technology and improvements in PV have made these sources very attractive to meet the energy needs of remote communities through a combination of wind turbine/battery storage/PV and backup diesel/generator systems.

This paper describes the design of a hybrid wind power storage and generation system and the electric power distribution system to provide the water and electric supply needs of a remote community.

16.2. Specifications and Constraints

For the purpose of this design, a farm community which comprises fifty (50) residents, with live stock of 40 cows, 10 steers, 30 pigs, 30 goats, 150 chicken and five 1000 square-foot garden plots for vegetables is considered. The electric supply system which should provide a fairly reliable, safe and economically justifiable source for pumping water and electric energy for lighting, heating, cooking and refrigeration of perishable goods and medical supplies. As a critical case of no wind for three days in a week, the system should be able to provide "critical load" for reserve potable (suitable for drinking) water supply and the necessary electric power for minimal lighting and refrigeration of medical supplies and perishable food items. The average wind speed at this location is assumed to be 14 miles per hour (class 3 site).

Some of the constraints include that the largest wind turbine size available is 10 kW. The battery must be sized to meet the peak and fluctuating load requirements while being only sixty percent efficient. Also the battery should not be depleted beyond twenty (20%) percent of its storage capacity. The diesel/generator is considered to be only 80% efficient and must be able to meet the emergency load demand. The total cost of the system should not exceed $500,000. PV is not considered to be a viable source at this location.

The projected daily water supply need of the community at the end of 25 years is shown in Table 16.1. The requirement for a reserve of drinkable water supply in the case of no wind for a three (3) day period is met through a storage tank of 122 cubic meters capacity. A 1.5 kW electric motor/submersible water pump was selected to meet the daily water requirements and to provide sufficient storage. The water well is assumed to be 230 ft or (70 m) deep with a static water level of 184 feet (56 m).

Table 16.1: Community Daily Water Usage Requirement.[7]

Description	Consumption Rate	Total Use (in Liters)	Future (in Liters)
Dairy Cattle (40)	70 Liter	2,800	4,000
Steers (10)	60 Liter	600	985
Pigs (30)	20 Liter	600	985
Goats (30)	10 Liter	300	492
Chickens (150)	0.3 Liter	45	74
Bathtub/Filing	130 Liter	6,500	10,670
Flush Toilet	10 Liter	500	820
Dish Washing/day	80 Liter	4,000	6,564
Laundry	190 Liter	9,500	15,586
Misc. Uses	90 Liter	4,500	7,385
Gardens	2,270 Liter	11,350	18,625
Total Water Usage		40,695	66,786

The power demand ratings for various appliances used in this study are given in Table 16.2.

Table 16.2: Power Demand for Various Appliances

Device Description	Demand (kW)/Device
Compact Fluorescent Lamp	0.015
Space Heater	1.500
15 ft^3 Frost-Free Freezer	0.114
20 ft^3 Frost-Free Freezer	0.114
Electric Cooking Range	1.250
Electric Oven	1.330
Washing Machine	0.250

The total numbers of various appliances used by the whole community include; 35 - compact fluorescent lights (CFL), 13 - electric stoves, 19 - electric space heaters, 13 - 15 ft^3 frost-free freezers, one - 20 ft^3 frost-free freezer, 6 - washing machines, 13 - electric ovens and one submersible water pump with a 1.5 kW motor. Knowing the total numbers of each type of appliance in use, and the rating of the appliance, the total diversified demand per appliance is then calculated. Using the hourly variation factor for each appliance, the numbers of appliances, the total load for that hour is calculated through an accumulation of each load.[8] Because of lack of actual load data this hourly load data is used as the peak load curve for the community. This load is then projected for the next twenty-five (25) years at a growth rate of two percent (2%) and is shown in Figure 16.1.

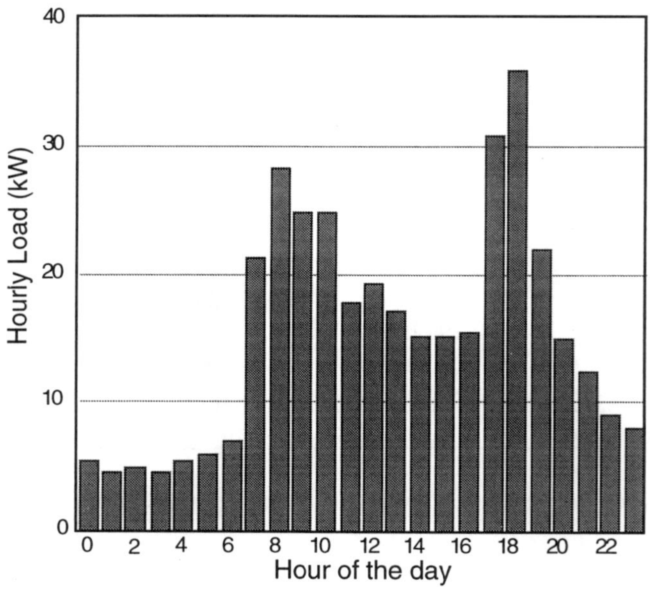

Figure 16.1. Projected community daily load profile.

16.3. Alternatives Considered and Selection of A Proposed Design

Because of the assumptions and constraints specified earlier, only wind turbines and wind turbines in combination with battery storage and backup diesel generator system were considered. None of the other renewable energy sources were considered because they were not available at this location.

Considering that the maximum demand is only 36 kW and it occurs at 6:00 pm., the following eight different alternatives consisting of wind power as the main source of energy but with various sizes of storage battery and backup diesel generator systems were considered.

An additional constraint in the selection of a cost effective design was that it provide the minimum power for lighting, and refrigeration of perishable food items and medicine even during the **worst case** scenario of the system not having wind power for three consecutive days any time during the year.

The fixed and operating costs of each design are tabulated in Table 16.3 along with the annualized costs over the 25 years at an interest rate of eight (8%) percent. This provides the basis for the selection from among various alternatives. The "worst case" requirement eliminated most of the wind only design alternatives. Based upon minimum annual cost over the 25 year period, design #8 was selected as the most cost effective.

Table 16.3: Alternate Designs Considered

Alternative	Description
Design 1.	5 - 10 kW Wind turbines
Design 2.	4 - 10 kW and 5 - 1.5 kW Wind turbines.
Design 3.	4 - 10 kW Wind turbines and 1-10 kW Diesel Generator.
Design 4.	3 - 10 kW Wind turbines and 1-25 kW Diesel Generator.
Design 5.	3 - 10 kW Wind turbines, 1 - 1.5 kW wind turbine and 1 - 120 kWh Storage battery.
Design 6.	4 - 10 kW Wind turbines, 1 - 100 kWh storage battery.
Design 7.	4 -10 kW Wind turbines, 1 - 30 kWh Storage battery, and 1 - 10 kW Diesel Generator.
Design 8.	3 - 10 kW wind turbine, 30 kWh Storage battery, and 1 - 17.5 kW Diesel Generator.

Table 16.4: Capital, Operating and Annual Costs of Design Alternatives

Design Alternative	Capital Cost	O&M Cost	Fuel Cost	Annual Cost
Design # 1.	115,220	1,047	0	11,841
Design # 2.	136,532	1,241	0	14,031
Design # 3.	94,319	916	1,405	11,157
Design # 4.	72,853	1,182	6,599	14,606
Design # 5.	102,663	933	0	10,550
Design # 6.	111,920	1,017	0	11,502
Design # 7.	100,920	987	318	10,758
Design # 8.	78,903	1,228	1,675	10,294

16.4. Design of Electric Distribution System

Next step is the design of an electric distribution system to provide power to each individual building in the community. The most favorable location for the wind turbine system was two miles away from the community center. One of the constraint in the design is that the maximum voltage drop allowed is five (5%) percent at any point of the system from the source. The selected distribution system design consists of a 3-phase, 7,200/240-120 step up transformer, a two mile long, #336,400 ACSR primary feeder, 2 - 10 kVA, four 25 kVA volt step down distribution transformers and service drops to individual loads.

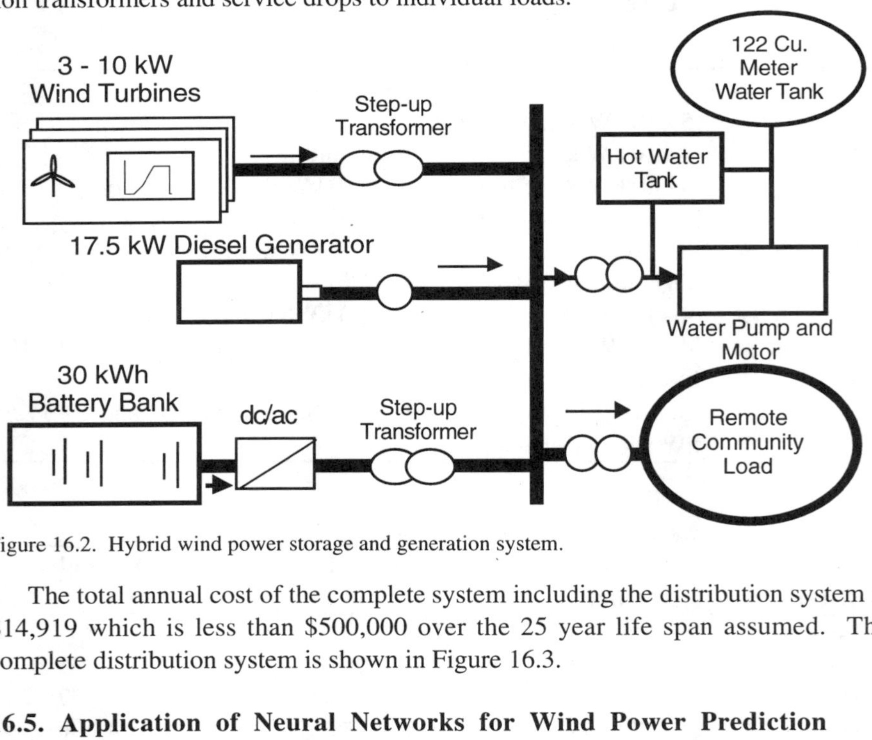

Figure 16.2. Hybrid wind power storage and generation system.

The total annual cost of the complete system including the distribution system is $14,919 which is less than $500,000 over the 25 year life span assumed. The complete distribution system is shown in Figure 16.3.

16.5. Application of Neural Networks for Wind Power Prediction

Available wind sources in the US could provide up to 10% of its energy needs. However, one of the reasons for low level of wind energy penetration into the generation mix is the lack of prediction of the wind power available at any time interval. A knowledge of available power over the next time interval of one hour, one day and even a month is very useful for operational control and generation scheduling. So it is important that a reliable tool to predict the availability of wind power over the next interval, an hour, next 24 hours, or a month be available. Neural networks have proven themselves to be very fast, reliable and fault-tolerant especially for pattern recognition, function approximation, and non-linear prediction.

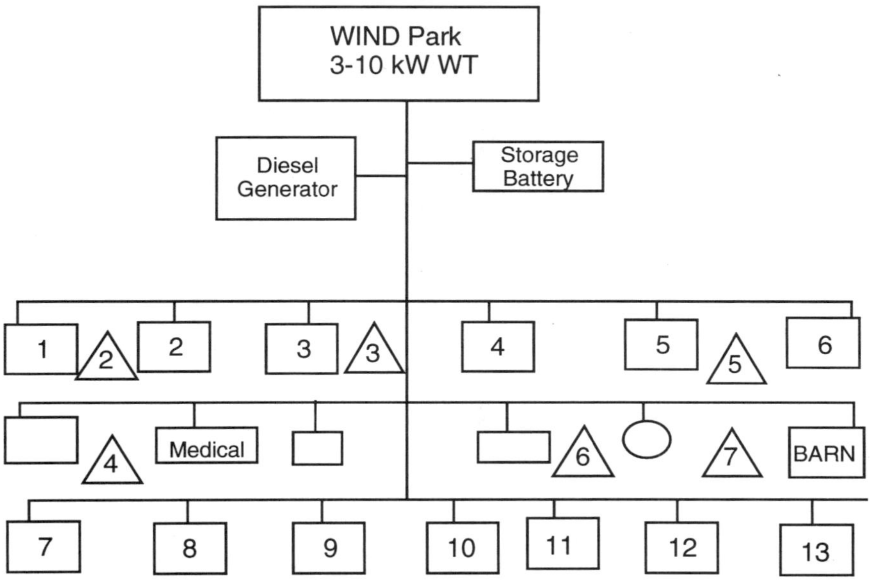

Figure 16.3. Power distribution system for the community.

In our effort to develop a suitable Artificial Neural Network (ANN) architecture for predicting wind power available over several time intervals, we have used back-propagation based feed forward neural networks with single and double hidden layers and with different numbers of neuron in each layer. The wind data used in training was taken from the HYBRID I software provided by University of Massachusetts. The total data is 720 points for one month at one hour intervals. The data was first normalized and a portion of it was used for training the network and some of the other part of the data was used for testing the performance of the predictor. Figure 16.4 shows a neural network configuration and iterative prediction structure where the network is given an initial set of past data and it produces the predicted future values by iterating the output back into the input of the network. Figure 16.5 shows the actual and neural network-based predicted values of 10 next data points using single hidden layer architecture. The network had 10 neuron in the first layer, 20 neuron in hidden layer and one in the output layer. Figure 16.6 shows prediction results using a two hidden layer network. But this is different from Figure 16.5 because only one data point is predicted at a time. This network had 4 neuron in first layer, 6 in first hidden layer and 10 in second hidden layer. The difference in actual and predicted data is in normalized form.

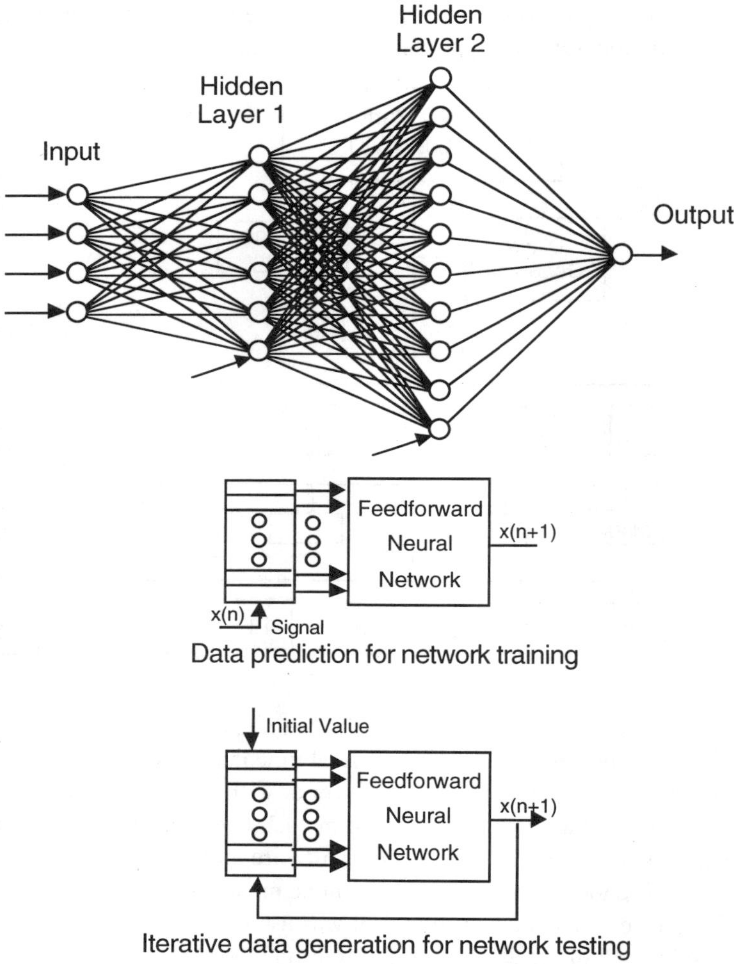

Figure 16.4. Neural network configuration and interative predictive structure.

16.6. Conclusions and Recommendations

This was a very good design project for an undergraduate student and provided the student an appreciation of the renewable energy sources as a viable alternative to meet the energy needs of remote communities in developed and under-developed countries. The neural network prediction work is continuing for further development of an optimum architecture.

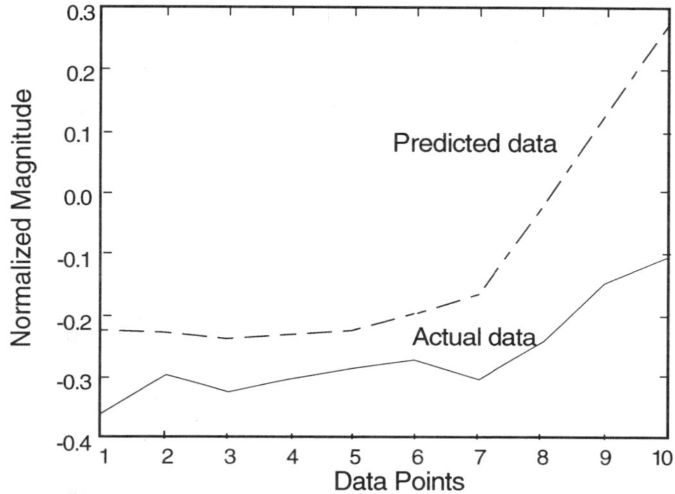

Figure 16.5. Prediction of 10 data points for training of 300 points (10-20).

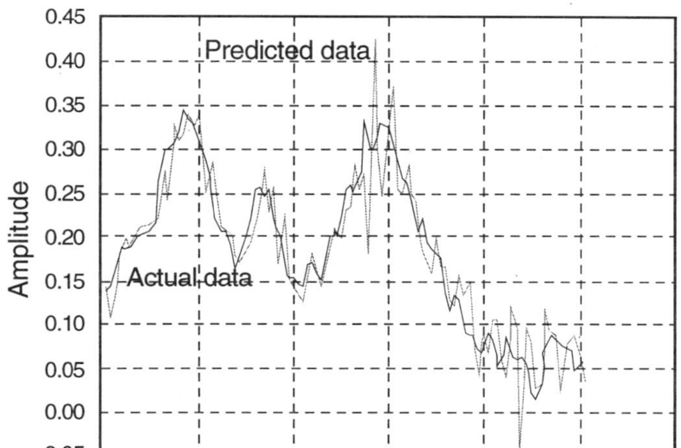

Figure 16.6. Prediction for 100 data points for training of 300 points (4-6-10).

16.7. Acknowledgment

The authors appreciate the support provided by the U.S. Department of Energy's National Renewable Energy Laboratory (NREL) under sub-contract Number XAH-3-13203-01 which funded the student's work.

16.8. References

1. A.H.M.S. Ula, "Global warming and electric power generation - What is the connection?," *IEEE Trans. on Energy Conversion* **6(4)** (December 1991).
2. EPA.430-R-94-001, "Energy Efficiency and Renewable Energy," (U.S. Environmental Protection Agency, Feb. 1994).
3. T. Beardsley, "Hot Air," *American Scientific* (September 1994) 18.
4. Gerhard Ott, "Energy demand, the environment, and population growth," *Siemens Review* **60** (March/April 1993) 34-37.
5. T. Beardsley "Turning Green," *American Scientific* (September 1994) 96-97.
6. Frank R. Eldridge, *Wind machines*, second edition (Van Nostrand Reinhold Company, New York, 1980).
7. P. Gipe, *Wind power for home and business: Renewable energy for the 1990 and beyond* (Chelsea Green Publishing Company, Post Mills, Vermont, 1993), pp. 257.
8. T. Gonen, *Electric Power Distribution System Engineering* (McGraw-Hill, Inc., New York, NY, 1986), pp. 62-63.

17. THE IMPORTANCE OF ARTIFICIAL NEURAL NETWORKS IN BIOMEDICINE

HARRY B. BURKE, M.D., PH.D.
Department of Medicine, New York Medical College
Valhalla, New York 10595, USA
E-mail: burke@unr.edu

ABSTRACT

The future explanatory power in biomedicine will be at the molecular-genetic level of analysis (rather than the epidemiologic-demographic or anatomic-cellular levels). This is the level of complex systems. Complex systems are characterized by nonlinearity and complex interactions. It is difficult for traditional statistical methods to capture complex systems because traditional methods attempt to find the model that best fits the statistician's understanding of the phenomenon; complex systems are difficult to understand and therefore difficult to fit with a simple model. Artificial neural networks are nonparametric regression models. They can capture any phenomena, to any degree of accuracy (depending on the adequacy of the data and the power of the predictors), without prior knowledge of the phenomena. Further, artificial neural networks can be represented, not only as formulae, but also as graphical models. Graphical models can increase analytic power and flexibility. Artificial neural networks are a powerful method for capturing complex phenomena, but their use requires a paradigm shift, from exploratory analysis of the data to exploratory analysis of the model.

17.1. Introduction

In the past, most biomedical phenomena were analyzed at the demographic-epidemiologic or anatomic-cellular levels. Since phenomena at these levels is largely linear or nearly linear, traditional statistical models were very helpful. One result of these analyses is that, today, most biomedical variables are linear or nearly linear variables. But the future will not be like the past. The future explanatory power in biomedicine is at the molecular-genetic level of analysis. This level is characterized by complex systems, i.e., nonmonotonicity (the outcome probability, in terms of the variable, is not constantly increasing or decreasing, for example, nonlinearity) and complex interactions. Complex systems are difficult for traditional statistical models to capture because traditional methods require a priori information about the variables in order to represent the variables in the model. Thus, the traditional statistician must "explore" the data, and must explicitly model what is discovered. But exploration

†This research was supported by the U.S. Army Medical Research and Development Command, Breast Cancer Research Program (DAMD 17-94-J-4383).

and explicit modeling is not always practical at the molecular-genetic level, where there can be twenty or more variables, and where the variables may interact in three-way and higher combinations.

There is evidence that cancer is a complex system and that future prognostic factors will be nonmonotonic and exhibit complex interactions. Cancer is primarily a genetic disease (Fearon 1990, Fishel *et. al.* 1993, Leach *et. al.* 1993) and a complex system. Cancer genes do not act in isolation; oncogenes, suppressor genes, and genetic mutations cause cancer through the complex interaction of the genes and their products (Papadopoulos *et. al.* 1994, Steel 1993). A cascade of genetic abnormalities is required to produce a cancer (Knudson 1985, Fearon and Vogelstein 1990). Thus, it cannot be assumed (1) that a gene or its product will be monotonic or that it will have an independent prognostic value before it is combined with other genes and/or their products, (2) that gene interactions are binary, or (3) that there will only be a few simple genetic interactions. Furthermore, it will probably not be possible to specify in advance of the analysis which complex genetic interactions exist. The need to capture nonmonotonicity and complex interactions exists because the prognostic value of the genetic changes and their products can depend on their nonmonotonic characteristics and interactions (Fearon and Vogelstein 1990).

17.2. Artificial Neural Networks

Artificial neural networks are a class of nonlinear regression and discrimination statistical methods, and they are of proven value in many areas of medicine (Westenskow *et. al.* 1992, Tourassi *et. al.* 1993, Leong and Jabri 1992, Palombo 1992, Gabor and Seyal 1992, Goldberg *et. al.* 1992, O'Leary *et. al.* 1992, Dawson *et. al.* 1991, Wu *et. al.* 1993, Astin and Wilding 1992, Weinstein *et. al.* 1992). In medical research, the most commonly used artificial neural networks are multilayer perceptrons that use backpropagation training. Backpropagation consists of fitting the parameters (weights) of the model by a criterion function, usually square error or maximum likelihood, using a gradient optimization method. In backpropagation artificial neural networks, the error is propagated back from the output to the connection weights in order to adjust the weights in the direction of minimum error. Artificial neural networks are usually composed of three interconnected layers of nodes: an input layer, a hidden layer, and an output layer, with each input node corresponding to a patient variable. All nodes after the input layer sum the inputs to them and use a transfer function (also known as an activation function) when they send the information to the adjacent layer nodes. The transfer function is usually a sigmoid function such as the logistic. The connections between the nodes have adjustable weights that specify the extent to which the output of one node will be reflected in the activity of the adjacent layer nodes. These weights, along with the connections among the nodes, determine the output of the network.

The mathematical representation of a multilayer perceptron (artificial neural network) can be viewed as a series of regression equations within a regression equation, where there can be as many regression equation as is necessary to fit the phenomenon. Thus,

$$h_j = f(w^h_{j1}x_1 + w^h_{j2}x_2 + \cdots + w^h_{jn}x_n) \tag{17.1}$$

$$o_j = g(w^o_1 h_1 + w^o_2 h_2 + \cdots + w^o_n h_n) \tag{17.2}$$

h_j in Eq. (17.1) is the output of each of the hidden nodes j, f is a nonlinear transfer function, w^h is the weight from predictor i to hidden node j, and x_i is an input variable. o_j in Eq. (17.2) is the prediction of the network, g is a nonlinear transfer function, w^o is the weight to the output node, and h is the hidden node output. It should be noted that Eq. (17.2), without Eq. (17.1) input, is equivalent to logistic regression, where g is the logistic function, w is the beta coefficient, and h is the x covariate. Artificial neural networks with sufficient hidden units can approximate any continuous function to any degree of accuracy (Hornik *et. al.* 1989, Leshno *et. al.* 1993).

17.3. Clinical Example

We have compared the prognostic accuracy of the TNM staging system (Beahrs *et. al.* 1992) and an artificial neural network according to five year cancer-specific survival.

Data. We have used three data sets in these analyses: two from the American College of Surgeon, the Patient Care Evaluation (PCE) breast cancer and colorectal cancer data sets; the National Cancer Institute's Surveillance, Epidemiology, and End Results (SEER) breast cancer data set; and the Mayo Clinic prostate cancer data set. The variables in the PCE, SEER, and Mayo data sets are either binary or monotonic. The factors were selected in the past for collection because they were significant in a generalized linear model, e.g., logistic regression. There is no predictive model that can improve upon a generalized linear model when the predictor variables meet the assumptions of the model and there are no interactions.

Accuracy. There are three components to predictive accuracy: the quality of the data, the predictive power of the prognostic factors, and the prognostic method's ability to capture the power of the prognostic factors. This work focuses on the third component. Comparative accuracy is assessed by the area under the receiver operating characteristic curve (Hanley and McNeil 1982). The receiver operating characteristic area varies from zero to one. When the prognostic score is unrelated to survival, the score is 0.5, indicating chance accuracy. The farther the score is from 0.5 the stronger the prediction model. Specifically, the TNM staging system's predictive accuracy is determined by comparing (using the area under the ROC curve) its prediction for each individual patient, where the prediction is the fraction of all the patients in that stage who survive, to each patient's true outcome.

Model. The artificial neural network results reported in this paper are based on backpropagation training which uses the maximum likelihood criterion function and the gradient descent optimization method and the "NevProp" software implementation for training. Significant differences in the receiver operating characteristic areas between the TNM staging system and the artificial neural network are tested following Hanley and McNeil (1982). The training data set is divided into training and stop-training subsets. Training is stopped when accuracy starts to decline on the stop-training data subset. All analyses employ the same training and testing (validation) data sets, and all results are based on the one time use of the testing data sets.

Results. A comparison of the accuracy of the TNM staging system and the artificial neural network (Table 17.1) using the PCE breast cancer data set, which examines breast cancer-specific five-year survival accuracy for only the TNM variables, demonstrates that the artificial neural network's predictions are significantly more accurate (TNM 0.720 vs. ANN 0.770, $p < 0.001$). Adding 51 commonly collected variables to the TNM variables further increases the accuracy of the artificial neural network (0.784). Extending these results to the SEER breast cancer data set, with a breast cancer-specific ten year survival endpoint; using only the TNM variables, the artificial neural network's prognostic accuracy is significantly greater than the TNM staging system (TNM 0.692 vs. ANN 0.730, $p < 0.01$).

Table 17.1: Comparison of TNM staging system and artificial neural networks (all comparisons are for five year, cancer-specific survival).

Data Sets	TNM	ANN
PCE 1983 Breast Cancer - TNM v	.720	.770
PCE 1983 Breast Cancer - 54 v	.720	.784
SEER 1977 Breast Cancer - TNM v, 10 yr	.692	.730
PCE 1983 Colorectal Cancer - TNM v	.737	.815
PCE 1983 Colorectal Cancer - 87 v	.737	.869
Mayo Clinic Prostate Cancer	.563	.811

Using the PCE colorectal data sets, the predictive accuracy of the two methods can be compared. For only the TNM variables, the artificial neural network's prognostic accuracy is significantly greater than the TNM stage model in predicting colorectal-specific five year survival (TNM 0.737 vs. ANN 0.815, $p < 0.001$). Adding 84 commonly collected factors to the TNM variables further increases the accuracy of the artificial neural network (0.869).

The Mayo Clinic data set demonstrates that, for prostate cancers represented in its corpus, the TNM staging system has a low prognostic accuracy (0.563), and that the artificial neural network, with other commonly collected variables, is significantly more accurate (TNM 0.563 vs. ANN 0.811, $p < 0.001$).

17.4. The Future of Artificial Neural Networks

To demonstrate the power of the artificial neural network to capture unanticipated nonmonotonicities and complex interactions, a constructed nonmonotonic variable is added to the 54 PCE breast cancer variables. The constructed nonmonotonic variable consists of two normal distributions centered at zero, one having a standard deviation of 1 for patients who are alive at five years, the other having a standard deviation of 10 for patients who are dead by five years. If the artificial neural network cannot capture nonmonotonicity without a priori specification of the phenomena, then its accuracy should remain at 0.770 with the TNM variables and 0.784 with the 54 variables, on the test set. The artificial neural network does capture the predictive power of the nonmonotonic factor, and its accuracy increases to 0.948 with the TNM variables and to 0.961 with the 54 variables, on the test set (Table 17.2).

Table 17.2: PCE 1983 Breast Cancer Data: 5 year Survival Prediction Accuracy, nonmonotonic variable added or three-way interaction added.

	nonmonotonic variable		three-way
Prediction Model	**TNM variables accuracy***	**55 variable accuracy***	**57 variable accuracy***
pTNM Stages	.720	.720	.720
Stepwise Logistic Regression	.762	.776	.776
Backpropagation ANN	.948	.961	.942

* The area under the curve of the receiver operating characteristic.

A constructed complex three-way interaction is added to the 54 PCE breast cancer variables. The artificial neural network captures the informative three-way interaction, from among the 29,260 possible three-way interactions, its accuracy increases from 0.784 to 0.942 on the test data set. It is the case that anticipated nonmonotonicity has, with varying degrees of success, been modeled by classical prediction models. Although it is computationally intensive, classical prediction models can test for a predictive three-way interaction among 29,260 possibilities, but it is not clear how they would discover four-way and higher interactions of nonlinear variables. It can be concluded that artificial neural networks are powerful models; they can capture the explanatory power inherent in complex systems.

At the present time, using variables selected by traditional statistical methods, it is not required that an artificial neural network be more accurate than traditional statistical methods in order for it to be an appropriate statistical method for cancer prediction. Artificial neural networks can be recommended for cancer prediction because: (1) they are as accurate as the best traditional statistical methods (Burke *et. al.*), (2) they are able to capture complex phenomena (e.g., nonmonotonicity and complex interactions) without a priori knowledge, and (3) they are a general regression method, therefore, if the phenomenon is not complex, so that accuracy can be maintained using a simpler model, artificial neural networks can be reduced to simpler models resulting in simpler representations.

There are several possible objections to artificial neural networks, including: (1) they require an analysis of the model. They capture phenomena without requiring prior exploration of the data, but they require exploration of the model. More will be said regarding model analysis later in the paper. (2) Some believe that artificial neural networks are overparameterized because they can have a large number of weights. Overfitting can be prevented by keeping the weights small, thereby reducing the effective number of degrees of freedom. This can be accomplished by penalizing large weights, or stopping the iterative fitting algorithm before the weights have grown to their full size. It is often the case that, when one of these methods is used, predictive accuracy is better than it would be if we used a smaller model and fit the data without restriction. When a method is used that reduces the weights that are not being increased by the input variables, the weights to the hidden layer shrink, and when there are only linear relationships present, as the hidden layer weights approach zero the neural network approximates a generalized linear model.

(3) It is thought that artificial neural networks are less "transparent" (the importance of the variables is less obvious), than traditional statistical models. This view of transparency fundamentally misunderstands the situation. Artificial neural networks are as complex as is necessary to capture the phenomenon. Generally, if the phenomenon is complex, the model must be complex. If the phenomenon is simple enough to be captured by simple models, then artificial neural networks can be reduced to a simple model, and the importance of covariates is easily observed. For example, if the phenomenon is linear, then a two layer (no hidden layer) artificial neural network with linear transfer functions, is mathematically identical to linear regression, and the weights of the artificial neural network are identical to the beta coefficients of the linear regression model. Therefore, model transparency (i.e., ease of variable interpretation) is properly understood as a function of complexity and

accuracy. For a simple phenomena, a properly chosen simple model is easily interpretable. For a complex phenomenon (e.g., complex interactions) and a properly chosen model, increases in model complexity result in increases in accuracy if overfitting is avoided. Increases in model complexity reduce the transparency of both traditional statistical models and artificial neural network statistical models.

17.5. Domain Knowledge and Model Knowledge

Domain knowledge is information regarding the phenomena acquired by examining the data, model knowledge is information regarding the phenomena acquired by examining the empirically derived model. Both are required for understanding phenomena, but their relative importance in the overall analysis can differ. In traditional statistics domain knowledge is the dominant approach. The statistician talks to the researcher, who suggests where the statistician can explore the data. The statistician then examines the data, finds the best fitting model, and performs inferential calculations to determine variable significance and importance. But this is not the only possible approach to understanding phenomena. Selection of the best (most accurate predictions) model can be based on either knowing the relationships between the predictors and the relationship of the predictors to the phenomenon, and selecting the model that best captures these relationships, or, if the relationships are not known a priori, selecting a model that is capable of capturing any relationships. This latter approach, selecting the model that can capture any phenomena, is very different from the traditional approach. It requires that the model be explored rather than the data. The relationships are captured in the model, and one decomposes the model in order to discover the phenomena.

It should be noted that, in terms of models, there is no difference between prediction and classification. Prediction and classification differ in the questions being asked, i.e., the character of the data and the type of outcome. Thus robotic control, from a model theoretic perspective, does not differ from cancer outcome prediction: vision is classification and movement is prediction.

There are some aspects of the analysis of a phenomena that are domain specific, and some that are model specific. For example, the number of hidden layer nodes (i.e., subregression equations) is domain specific. The number of hidden layer units cannot be determined, a priori, by any analytic method because the number of units depends on the complexity of the phenomena; a simple phenomena requires no hidden units, a complex may require five or ten hidden units.

An example of model analysis is the determination of whether the phenomenon exhibits nonmonotonicities or complex interactions. The approach is to compare the results of a two-layer neural network with those of a three-layer neural network. If the two-layer is significantly less accurate than the three-layer neural network, then there are nonmonotonic relationships, interactions, or both. If there is no difference between the two models, then the model can be simplified. If there is a difference, then a complex (three-layer) model must be used to capture the nonlinearities and interactions.

For simple phenomena, e.g., phenomena that do not require the use of a hidden layer in an artificial neural network, artificial neural networks are as transparent as other statistical models. For complex models sensitivity analysis can determine the contribution of input variables in the artificial neural network prediction (Intrator 1993). But sensitivity analysis is not adequate because complex relationships, represented by complex mathematical equations, are not easily understood. To understand these complex relationships visual models are needed. Buntine (1994) points out "Graphical operations manipulate the underlying structure of a problem unhindered by the fine detail of the connecting functional and distributional equations. This structuring process is important in the same way that a high-level programming language leads to higher productivity over assembly language."(p 160) The ability to represent and manipulate artificial neural networks, in terms of graphical models, provides power and flexibility in model analysis.

17.6. References

Astin M.L., Wilding P., "Application of neural networks to the interpretation of laboratory data in cancer diagnosis," *Clin. Chem.* **38** (1992) 34-38.

Beahrs O.H., Henson D.E., Hutter R.V.P., Kennedy B.J., *Manual for staging of cancer*, 4th ed. (JB Lippincott, Philadelphia, PA, 1992).

Buntine W.L., "Operations for learning with graphical models," *J. Art. Intell. Res.* **2** (1994) 159-225.

Burke H.B., Rosen D.B., Goodman P.H., "Comparing the prediction accuracy of artificial neural networks and other statistical models for breast cancer," *Advances in Neural Information Processing Systems 7,* ed.s G. Tesauro, D.S. Touretsky, and T.K. Leen (MIT Press, Cambridge, MA, 1995), pp. 1063-67.

Dawson A.E., Austin R.E., Weinberg DS., "Nuclear grading of breast carcinoma by image analysis," *J. Clin. Pathol.* **95**(Suppl) (1991) S29-S37.

Fearon E.R., Vogelstein B., "A genetic model for colorectal cancer," *Cell* **61**(1990) 759-67.

Fishel R., Lescoe M.K., Rao M.R.S., *et. al.*, "The human mutator gene homolog *MSH2* and its association with hereditary nonpolyposis colon cancer," *Cell* **75** (1993) 1027-36.

Gabor A.J., Seyal M. "Automated interictal EEG spike detection using artificial neural networks," *Electroencephalogr. Clin. Neurophysiol.* **83** (1992) 271-80.

Goldberg V., Manduca A, Ewert D.L., "Improvement in specificity of ultrasonography for diagnosis of breast tumors by means of artificial intelligence," *Med. Phys.* **19** (1992) 1275-81.

Hanley J.A., McNeil B.J., "The meaning of the use of the area under the receiver operating characteristic (ROC) curve," *Radiology* **143** (1982) 29-36.

Hornik K., Stinchcombe M., White H., "Multilayer feedforward networks are universal approximators," *Neural Networks* **2** (1989) 359-66.

Intrator O., Intrator N., "Neural networks for interpretation of nonlinear models," in *Proceedings of the Statistical Computing Section* (American Statistical Society, San Francisco CA, 1993), pp. 244-9.

Knudson A.G. Jr., "Hereditary cancer, oncogenes, and antioncogenes,"*Cancer Res.* **45** (1985) 1437-43.

Leach F.S., Nicolaides N.C., Papadopoulos N., *et. al.*, "Mutations of a *mutS* homolog in hereditary nonpolyposis colorectal cancer," *Cell* **76** (1993) 1215-25.

Leong P.H., Jabri M.A., "MATIC - an intracardiac tachycardia classification system," *PACE* **15** (1992) 1317-31.

Leshno M., Lin V.Y., Pinkus A., Schocken S., "Multilayer feedforward networks with a nonpolynomial activation function can approximate any function," *Neural Networks* **6** (1993) 861-67.

O'Leary T.J., Mikel U.V., Becker R.L., "Computer-assisted image interpretation: use of a neural network to differentiate tubular carcinoma from sclerosing adenosis," *Modern. Pathol.* **5** (1992) 402-5.

Palombo S.R., "Connectivity and condensation in dreaming," *J. Am. Psychoanal. Assoc.* **40** (1992) 1139-59.

Papadopoulos N., Nicolaides N.C., Wei Y., *et. al.*, "Mutation of a *mutL* homolog in hereditary colon cancer," *Science* **263** (1994) 1625-29.

Steel M., "Cancer genes: complexes and complexities," *Lancet* **342** (1993) 754-5.

Tourassi G.D., Floyd C.E., Sostman H.D., Coleman R.E., "Acute pulmonary embolism: artificial neural network approach for diagnosis," *Radiology* **189** (1993) 555-58.

Weinstein J.N., Kohn K.W., Grever M.R., Viswanadham V.N., Rubenstein L.V., Monks A.P., "Neural computing in cancer drug development: predicting mechanism of action," *Science* **258** (1992) 447-51.

Westenskow D.R., Orr J.A., Simon F.H., "Intelligent alarms reduce anesthesiologist's response time to critical faults," *Anesthesiology* **77** (1992) 1074-9.

Wu Y., Giger M.L., Doi K., Vyborny C.J., Schmidt R.A., Metz C.E., "Artificial neural networks in mammography: application to decision making in the diagnosis of breast cancer," *Radiology* **187** (1993) 81-87.

18. ADAPTIVE LOGIC NETWORKS IN REHABILITATION OF PERSONS WITH INCOMPLETE SPINAL CORD INJURY

WILLIAM W. ARMSTRONG
Department of Computing Science, University of Alberta
Edmonton, Alberta, Canada T6G 2H1
E-mail: arms@cs.ualberta.ca

and

Dendronic Decisions Limited, 3624 - 108 Street, NW
Edmonton, Alberta, Canada T6J 1B4

ALEKSANDAR KOSTOV, RICHARD B. STEIN
Division of Neuroscience, University of Alberta
Edmonton, Alberta, Canada T6G 2H1

and

MONROE M. THOMAS
Dendronic Decisions Limited, 3624 - 108 Street, NW
Edmonton, Alberta, Canada T6J 1B4

ABSTRACT

Persons with incomplete spinal cord injury are generally at least partially paralyzed and are often unable to walk. Manually-controlled electrical stimulation has been used to act upon nerves or muscles to cause leg movement so such persons can achieve functional walking. They use crutches or a mobile walker for support, and initiate each stimulus by pressing a button. Artificial intelligence and machine learning techniques are now making it possible to automate the process of stimulus-initiation. Supervised training of an automatic system can be based on samples of correct stimulation given by the patient or by a therapist, accompanied by data from sensors indicating the state of the person's body and its relation to the ground during walking. A major issue is generalization, i.e. whether the result of training can be used for control at a later time or in somewhat different circumstances. As the possibilities grow for increasing the number and variety of sensors on a patient, and for easily implanting more numerous stimulation channels, the need is increasing for powerful learning systems which can automatically develop effective and safe control algorithms. This paper explains the foundations of adaptive logic networks, and illustrates how they have been used to develop an experimental walking prosthesis used in a laboratory setting. Successful generalization has been observed using parameters from training which took place up to several days earlier.

18.1. Introduction

Today it is possible to apply advanced mechanical, electronic and computing technology to problems of rehabilitation of persons with spinal cord injury (SCI). One of the major thrusts has been in the area of functional electrical stimulation (FES) to cause paralyzed limbs to move and thereby restore a measure of walking capability (Stein 1993). One goal of using FES instead of a wheelchair is to be able to walk reasonably long distances and thereby provide a better blood supply to the paralyzed extremities. Another goal is to be mobile and independent in restricted spaces, such as in a kitchen or an ordinary bathroom where wheelchair access may be impossible. The most reliable method of control is using hand switches, but this is not appropriate for incomplete quadriplegics and stroke subjects who may not have adequate hand function. In addition, operating a hand switch requires repetitive voluntary intervention and can introduce delays and variability. Automatic control of FES is therefore desirable or necessary for some persons.

FES-aided walking is usually introduced into the rehabilitation program of selected spinal cord injured subjects in three distinct phases:

1. In the first phase, the subject has to increase the physical strength of his or her whole body, strength which has possibly been significantly reduced by hospitalization. The subject becomes familiar with basic FES principles and learns how an appropriate FES-system operates.
2. Standing with the appropriate mechanical aid (parallel bars, harness, frame, four-point walker) and fitted with the FES system, the subject learns how to operate the switch or switches to be used to start and stop stimulation. These are often mounted on the support aid.
3. The subject's gait training starts by extending the walking distance from a few steps between parallel bars to as many steps as he or she is comfortable with, using a mobile mechanical walking aid (a metal frame on wheels). A therapist will begin controlling the walk, but the patient is encouraged to take over as soon as possible.

Taking a step, which is an automatic process for people having normal voluntary control over their extremities, is a very complex process for someone whose extremities are paralyzed. In one case, to take a step, a subject with one completely and one only partially disabled leg has to perform twelve distinct actions to assure that her posture and the position of the walker produce a safe movement. The two most important and hazardous phases of this procedure are the shifts of weight to and from the disabled leg, and they usually take most of the subject's attention during walking, no matter which way the walking is controlled. These are the moments when it is not very clear to the subject which leg is in charge of supporting the main body weight.

Despite important advantages, manual control of FES has a few disadvantages. It doesn't provide the subject with the possibility of improving the quality of walking or of reaching distant points with less energy (efficiency of walking). Further improvement in locomotion requires stabilization of the stance phase and reduction in its duration, which can best be achieved by an automatic controller. The goal in designing an automatic control system for FES-assisted walking is to preserve or even improve the reliability and safety of a manual system, and to bring more functionality and more efficiency to the disabled gait. A major task in automating the control of walking for stroke or incomplete SCI subjects is to automatically recognize the intention to take a step with a disabled leg and to provide the required control signals to the stimulator.

Recognition can be based on physical measurements. An early means of automatic control in the case of foot drop used a heel switch which activated a single channel of stimulation to assist in the swing phase whenever the heel came off the ground. This simple system does not work reliably in subjects where contractures or spasticity prevent a good heel contact with sufficient weight bearing or in subjects who suffer from clonus (rapid contraction and relaxation of a muscle), which can cause the heel to lift and touch the ground several times during the stance phase. A rule-based system using threshold logic applied to the signal from a force sensor installed under the toe of the normal leg has been proposed as an alternative method to detect the subject's intention to take a step. The duration of the stimulation was either preset or it was determined by means of another force sensor installed under the toe of the stimulated leg.

The current study investigated automatic control of FES switching commands for straight-line walking based on the patterns of switching by a skilled subject or physiotherapist. Feedback as to the state of the body was derived through forces measured under the feet. The adaptive logic network (ALN), a type of artificial neural network, was used for supervised learning of the control. If the ALN could be trained to reproduce stimulation switching patterns, then the ALN could also be used to transform input sensory signals into output control signals for stimulation. This method is intended for subjects who are already trained to step periodically by manually pressing on a switch to turn stimulation on or off. Automatic control can then be added to manual control to enable the subject to concentrate on other functions during walking, such as shifting the body weight from one leg to another, avoiding obstacles, moving assistive devices, carrying objects, etc. Manual control or remaining capabilities after an incomplete SCI may be used to initiate and terminate walking.

At the present time, technology is advancing very rapidly in the areas of miniaturization and techniques for ease of implantation of sensors and stimulators. Many channels of information can be used at once to sense the state of a person's body and its relation to the ground, and many channels can be used to apply stimuli. The major problem is becoming one of controlling the stimuli as a function of sensor inputs, both present and past. This must be done not only with great economy of means, e.g. with a portable device that can cause complex patterns of stimulation, but it must ultimately be done without excessive cost for the individual's particular solution. Every case has to be handled on its own merits; for example there may be only partial paralysis of the legs, and a prosthesis can potentially use the remaining human sensory and motor capabilities to increase speed and stability, or to signal to the system that the person has the intention to take a step in a certain direction. Individualized development of hardware and software is very costly. Besides the initial development cost, any solution will likely have to be modified as the person changes, adapts and wishes to take on new challenges. Changes to the person's muscle tone, strength, tendency to fatigue, the presence of a temporary illness, and new challenges to mobility such as inclines or steps, will require changes to the control software.

A practical automatic FES control system is subject to constraints on size, weight, reliability, power consumption and cost. It must be fast enough for real-time operation, and permit upgrades when technology advances. In addition, the system must be such that, as far as possible, there will never be any unexpected stimuli generated: a sudden inappropriate stimulus could result in a serious fall. The cost factor suggests using inexpensive off-the-shelf components, while the need for real-time control means that a very efficient computational approach is required. In the following we report on a technique to automate FES control using adaptive logic networks (ALNs) that shows promise in solving these problems.

18.2. Adaptive Logic Networks

Artificial intelligence techniques, particularly artificial neural networks (Hecht-Nielsen 1990), offer hope for an effective solution for automatic control of FES in walking. A simple perceptron or linear threshold unit (LTU) accepts input vectors $(x_1, x_2, \ldots, x_n)$ having n real values as components, and outputs a Boolean value 1 if $w_0 + w_1x_1 + \ldots + w_nx_n \geq 0$. Otherwise it outputs 0. The sequence of weights $w_0, \ldots, w_n$ is called the weight vector of the LTU. The function computed by the LTU is determined by its weight vector. A neural net called a feedforward multilayer perceptron consists of a loop-free interconnection of units that typically form an inhomogeneous linear combination of their input signals $u = w_0 + w_1x_1 + \cdots + w_nx_n$ and pass this through a non-linearity of the form $\varphi(u) = 1/(1+e^{-u})$. The so-called input layer of the net just distributes input values to the next layer of units, the first hidden layer. There follow other hidden layers and an output layer. The reason for using a differentiable non-linearity in multilayer perceptrons instead of the hard limiter (the greater-than-or-equal-to operator used in the simple perceptron) was that no training procedure was known for the network of LTUs. The backpropagation training algorithm overcame this problem and multilayer perceptrons have been used successfully in solving control problems (Miller 1991).

In our study, ALNs provided the learning and execution power necessary. There have been, at various times, three quite distinct versions of the ALN concept:

1. Systems that learn Boolean functions by means of choosing functions AND, OR, LEFT or RIGHT at nodes of a fixed binary tree of flexible logic gates (Armstrong 1991).
2. Systems that encode real values into Boolean vectors by means of a variety of fixed thresholds on the real inputs, then submit those bit vectors to several systems of type 1 operating in parallel, and finally decode the resulting output bit vectors to produce a real value (Armstrong 1992, Armstrong 1993).
3. Systems which have LTUs with adaptive weights in the first hidden layer, and have only AND and OR gates in other hidden layers and the output layer (Armstrong 1994, Armstrong 1995).

The distinctive feature of all ALNs as compared to other multilayer perceptrons is their use of logic gates in all hidden layers but the first. Version 1 ALNs are generally unsuitable for FES applications because they are limited to Boolean inputs.

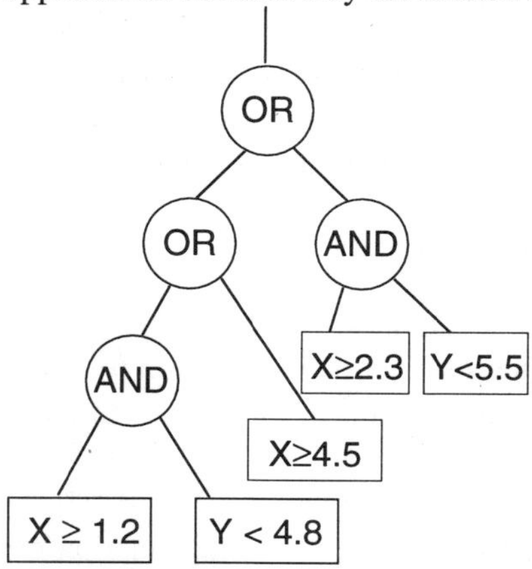

Figure 18.1. Structure of an ALN version 2 network. Note the use of fixed thresholds at the leaves.

ALN version 2 involves networks of logic gates whose inputs are computed by fixed thresholds on continuous input variables (sensor measurements). If a measurement value is greater than (or alternatively less than) a fixed threshold, then the input to the net is a logical 1, otherwise a 0. More complex schemes of encoding, in particular a technique for random walk encoding used in Atree 2.0 and 2.7

(Armstrong 1992) fail to preserve the monotonicity of the output signal as a function of input signals when it is desirable to make use of this property. An ALN version 2 is shown in Figure 18.1.

ALN version 2 networks adapt the functions at the nodes of the logic tree, which can be any of four kinds: AND, OR, LEFT and RIGHT. The last two, LEFT and RIGHT are the Boolean functions of two inputs whose outputs simply output the value on the specified left or right input of the node. After training is completed, all LEFT and RIGHT units are removed and replaced by the connections their function represents. Version 2 ALNs have been tested successfully for control (Supynuk 1992) and for FES applications (Kostov 1995a), however the complexity of encoding and decoding gives rise to doubts about their ease of understanding and hence their safety.

ALN version 3 involves using a logic network of ANDs and ORs with inputs from LTUs. An ALN version 3 network is shown in Figure 18.2.

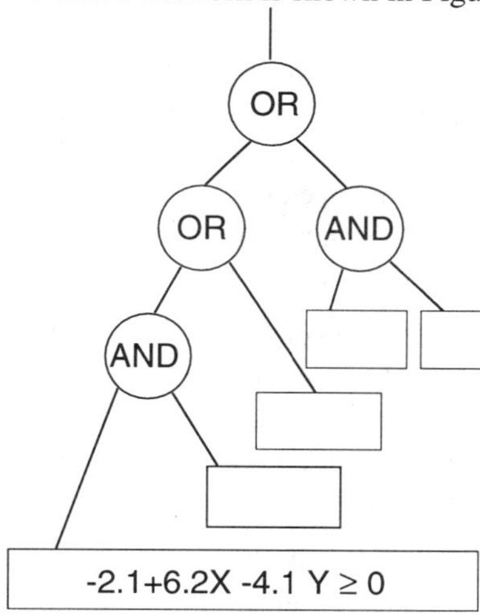

Figure 18.2. An ALN version 3 network.

Version 3 ALNs, though not capable of outputting real values, are capable of *representing* functions from reals to reals by classifying the set on and under the graph of a function as the 1-class and the rest of the inputs as the 0-class. Version 3 ALNs are just special cases of the earliest multilayer perceptrons where the units in hidden layers except the first are specialized to perform fixed Boolean logic operations AND and OR. Version 3 ALNs can be used in contexts where feedforward multilayer perceptrons are used. In addition, they can be used where additional knowledge is needed to constrain the properties of the learned function. ALN version 3 has been used in controlling a mechanical model of a vehicle active suspension system. (Armstrong 1994). The ease of inverting monotonic functions derived by ALN training was important in that application. The particular characteristics of functions synthesized by version 3 ALNs are as follows:

- ALNs allow arbitrary bounds on slopes (i.e. partial derivatives) to be imposed on functions during training. In particular, the learned function may be constrained to be weakly or strongly monotonic increasing (or decreasing) in any variable.
- The architecture of the logic tree can be used to impose qualitative constraints, such as convexity, on parts of learned functions. Qualitative *a priori* knowledge may be a result of general physical laws holding (conservation of energy, conservation of momentum, Le Chatelier's principle, etc.).
- Evaluation of the function represented by a trained ALN is done by a separate program and is very rapid. It is based on a decision tree DTREE which narrows down the computation for a particular input vector to involve as few as n linear computations, where n is the dimension of the space (including n -1 input variables and one output variable). The linear pieces are combined by maximum and minimum operations. Real-time bounds can be guaranteed even though the function graph may be made up of a very large number of linear pieces.
- There is no "black box." The behavior of a learned, piecewise linear function can be checked completely for conformity to a specification by examining all of the blocks of the input space determined by the decision tree and the simple combinations of linear pieces using maximum and minimum operations which compute the output in that block.
- The result of ALN training can be converted into a DTREE computation with a different output variable. A function inverse is obtained in this way. The variable must be one in which the original ALN output was forced to be monotonic.

The adaptation algorithm produces functions which are piecewise linear and continuous. We shall now illustrate how these arise, beginning with a one-LTU ALN in Figure 18.3.

The set of vectors which satisfy $w_0 + w_1 x_1 + \ldots + w_n x_n \geq 0$ will be referred to as the 1-set of the LTU (shown shaded in Figure 18.4 for the case $n = 2$). Its complement is the 0-set (the white area above the 1-set in Figure 18.4).

Since an LTU is unable to compute some simple functions, such as a function which is 1 inside a rectangle and 0 outside, it is natural to use multilayer networks composed of such units to increase the repertoire of computable functions. Then the inputs to layers after the LTUs are all Boolean, and the units at higher levels compute Boolean functions. We can see how an LTU could be used at a higher level in the net to compute an AND function. The value computed by the LTU would be 1 if and only if $-n + x_1 + x_2 + \ldots + x_n \geq 0$. An OR would be obtained by $-1 + x_1 + x_2 + \ldots + x_n \geq 0$. A negation, if required, could be computed by an LTU using the formula $0.5 - x_1 \geq 0$. Clearly ALNs version 3 are special cases of early multilayer perceptrons, though with a new training algorithm.

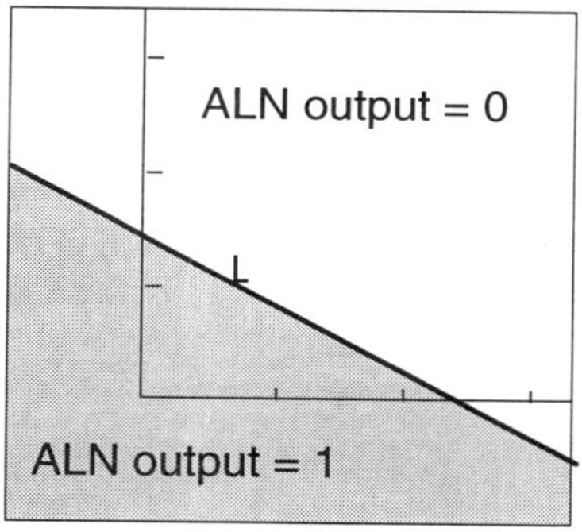

Figure 18.3. The half space under the line L: $1.4 - 0.57\,x - y = 0$.

During training of an ALN, there are changes to the weights of the LTUs. It is possible to allow changes to the logic functions at nodes of the tree, or to the architecture of the tree, but these will not be explored in this article since it was thought important for FES to have control over the qualitative properties of the synthesized function. Fixing the architecture and node functions of the logic tree allows one to constrain qualitative properties of the function to be learned. For example one can force it to be convex-up or convex-down.

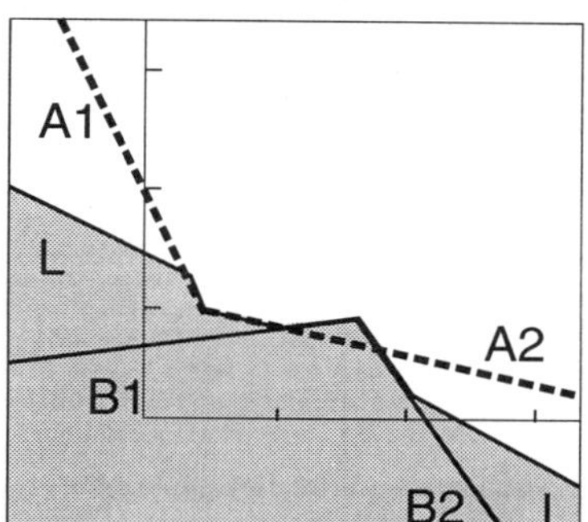

Figure 18.4. The shaded set of Figure 18.4 is the 1-set of the ALN shown in Figure 18.5.

The 1-set of an ALN is formed by taking unions and intersections (corresponding to OR and AND operations, respectively) of such half-spaces as are shown in Figure 18.3. In Figure 18.4 the shaded set of Figure 18.3 is intersected with the union of two half-spaces suggested by the dotted lines A1 and A2, and the union is taken with the intersection of two half-spaces as suggested by the solid lines B1 and B2. Note that the order of these two operations cannot be interchanged without cutting off a part of the shaded area.

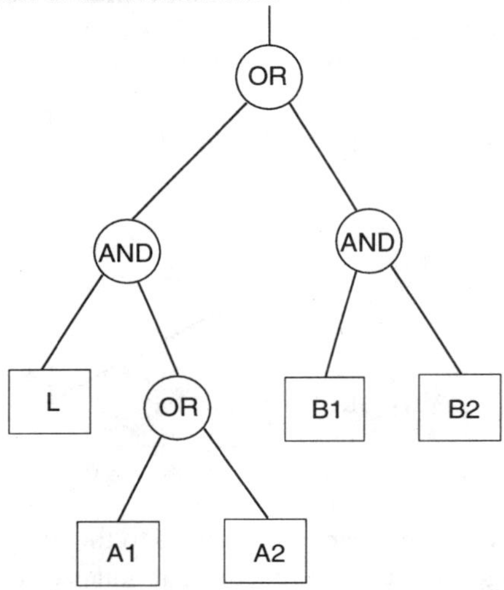

Figure 18.5. The ALN representing the shaded set in Figure 18.4.

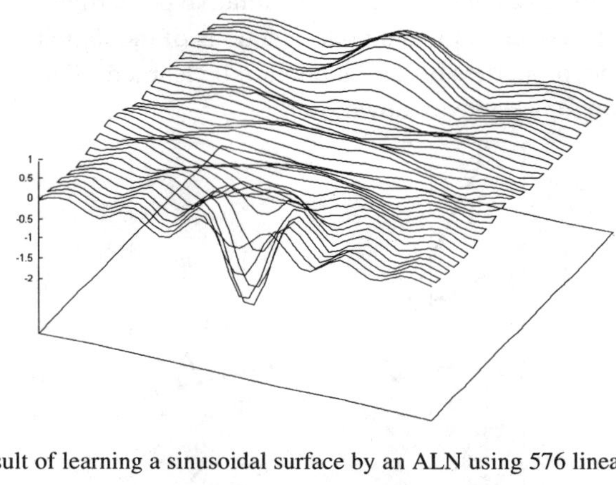

Figure 18.6. Result of learning a sinusoidal surface by an ALN using 576 linear pieces.

If a larger ALN is used, it is possible to approximate any continuous function to any precision uniformly on a compact set, as illustrated in Figure 18.6. The proof is quite simple: Riemann sums approximate the area under a continuous function, and the only modification which has to be made in a Riemann sum is to slant the edges of each pillar slightly so that a function is obtained which is represented by a two-layer ALN in the form of an OR of ANDs of linear functions. The weight on the output variable of each linear piece can be normalized to -1.

18.3. ALN training

The fundamental operation behind the adaptation of an LTU for an ALN is least-squares fitting of a collection of data points. The goal of adaptation is to determine weights that allow the LTU to separate vectors of the two classes. We are also going to use the LTU as a classifier, but the meaning of the classes will be quite unique to the ALN approach. Given a function, the 1-class will be defined as the set on and under the graph of the function. This is illustrated in Figure 18.7.

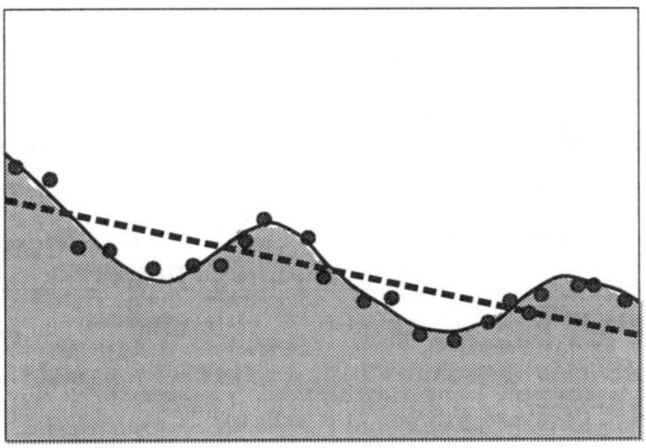

Figure 18.7. Fitting non-linear data with a single LTU.

The shaded part of Figure 18.7 represents a 1-class, and the part above the 0-class. In order to train a single LTU, a least-squares fitting algorithm is used (linear regression in statistical terminology). This training procedure supposes that we have a collection of points that represent function values, i.e. values on or near the *boundary* between the two classes. For example, in Figure 18.7, the dashed line shows a boundary between classes that might be estimated by linear regression.

In much of the work on the perceptron, it was trained not by giving points on the boundary between the classes, but by giving samples of the two classes, whether on the boundary or in the interior. In later work, the perceptron, fitted with a sigmoidal function, was used to approximate functions by means of its output. Networks of these units are a major force in neural network applications today. The work on ALNs has restored the use of the LTU as a classifier, and uses a network of LTUs and logic gates AND and OR to *represent* a piecewise linear function, but not to *compute* it directly.

We consider the situation when five LTUs are used to approximate the 1-set of the function in Figure 18.8. The logical expression for the 1-set according to these five lines is OR(L1, AND(L2, L3), AND(L4, L5)).

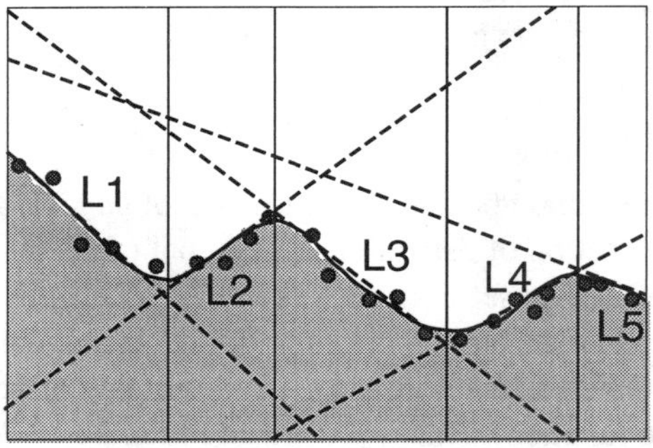

Figure 18.8. Fitting non-linear data with an ALN containing five LTUs.

The vertical lines in Figure 18.8 indicate the parts of the horizontal axis where each of the five lines is active. For example, L1 is active on the left end of the horizontal axis. The line L1 could be determined by linear regression on the leftmost five data points. Then L2 could be determined by the four points in the next interval, and so on. Performing a piecewise linear regression is well understood, and the only complication here is that as a linear piece moves to fit its data points, the very set of data points that belong to it may be exchanged with other linear pieces. ALN training is an iterative procedure which uses iterative methods to adjust the linear pieces computed by each LTU. It is recursively determined at each step which LTU is responsible for fitting the data point being presented to the net. Responsibility of an LTU is computed recursively from the root of the ALN tree based on the AND and OR gates at the nodes of the tree. For example, if two functions are represented by subtrees entering an AND gate, then the one which has the minimum value is the one which is responsible for the given data point.

18.4. Real-time Computation

If we look at the linear pieces as functions of the variable on the horizontal axis of Figure 18.8, we can write the function represented by this logical combination of LTUs as MAX(L1, MIN(L2, L3), MIN(L4, L5)). This "MIN/MAX" expression computes the function represented by the ALN on the whole space. To evaluate the MIN/MAX expression, it is possible to compute the values of all the linear pieces at a point and then evaluate the MIN/MAX expression shown. A much faster way will now be suggested. As shown in Figure 18.8, we take a partition of the horizontal axis as follows:

1. Divide the axis so that about half of the active line segments into which the curve is divided lie to the left, and half to the right.
2. Keep repeating the procedure for the resulting partitions until at most two linear pieces are active in any partition.

Figure 18.8 shows the horizontal axis divided into four partitions. Using this division scheme, at most two linear pieces are involved in the computation of the function in any division or block of the partition.

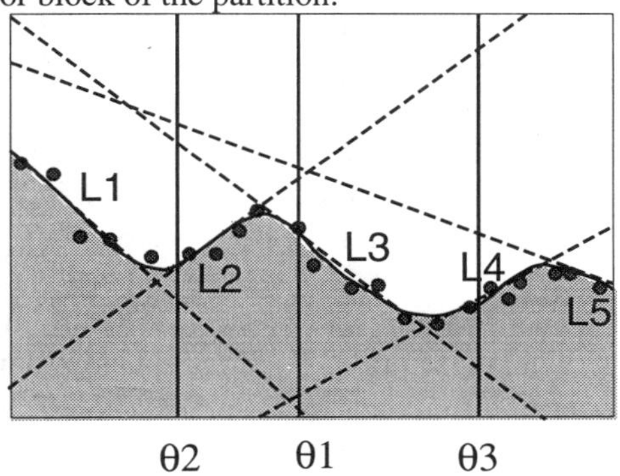

Figure 18.9. Partitioning the input space to reduce computation.

In the leftmost division we have to evaluate the expression MAX(L1, L2), in the next division MIN(L2, L3), in the next MAX(L3, L4), and finally MIN(L4, L5). The correct division is determined by a decision tree:

1. If $x < \theta_1$ then go to step 2. else go to step 3.
2. If $x < \theta_2$ then go to step 4 else go to step 5
3. If $x < \theta_3$ then go to step 6 else go to step 7.
4. Compute MAX(L1, L2).
5. Compute MIN(L2, L3).
6. Compute MAX(L3, L4).
7. Compute MIN(L4, L5).

The number of pieces in the partition ultimately depends on the complexity of the function being represented. At each comparison of the decision tree, the number of linear pieces that have to be evaluated drops by about half. In general, some pieces will cross the dichotomy, which makes the reduction less than half. Ultimately, the number of linear pieces in a division of the space is at most equal to the dimension of the space. If more pieces than the dimension of the space intersect at a point (giving an overdetermined solution to a system of linear equations), some pieces can be slightly perturbed to correct the situation. With this kind of hard bound on the number of linear pieces that have to be evaluated, it becomes possible to guarantee hard real-time bounds on the computation.

18.5. Training ALNs to Control FES

Many of the results reported below were obtained by A. Kostov (Kostov 1995). Two forms of ALN were used: ALN versions 2 and 3. For the application to FES, it is preferable to have an ALN structure that is composed of few linear pieces. One of the main reasons for this is the safety of the patient. A simple network, if it is adequate for the task of controlling a prosthesis, will be more easily understood by an expert who is checking the result of training. In addition, its operation will more quickly become familiar to the patient. In the case of one patient, a simple AND of several linear threshold elements was adequate for control, and the patient expressed satisfaction with the result. As inputs to the ALN, we have used the current measurements of force sensors at several points on insoles put into the patient's shoes, as well as several stored values which have been acquired a fixed interval of time earlier.

During a walking session, training data is accumulated from the sensors and the therapist's or patient's switching actions. The data is analyzed using ALN learning, a process requiring about thirty seconds on a 486DX2-50 PC, and then the learned functions, turned into decision trees, are ready for use in automatic control. Figure 18.10 shows traces of the force sensors in the shoes, the stimuli given manually, and the automatic stimuli obtained by replaying the original signals after ALN training.

The prosthesis is not entirely dependent on ALN learning for its operation. Restriction rules (RR) are used to prevent a stimulus being given in a situation where it might not be safe, for example in the case of clonus. The rules were implemented separately from the ALN, though it will be possible in future to implement them as part of the *a priori* knowledge constraining ALN training.

Restriction rules embody one type of a priori knowledge that can be used to constrain the system. Other types of expert knowledge could be used as is done when using the fuzzy set concept for control. *Fuzzy control* often uses piecewise linear functions like the ALN, the difference being that a designer can express information about measurements in the form of linguistic terms. For example, it might be a requirement to take a certain action when the pressure on the left heel is "high." The extent to which pressure is high could be represented by a piecewise linear function with values between 0 and 1. We feel that fuzzy control ideas could be valuable in setting up ALNs initially, based on expert knowledge, and the initial state would be changed by ALN training to better reflect empirical data.

ALNs were evaluated for cloning the manual skill of a skilled subject or therapist in controlling one channel of stimulation for FES-assisted walking. The capability of ALNs to generate control rules from manually controlled stimulation was demonstrated. In addition, it was demonstrated that the quality of ALN learning depends on the number of sensory feedback channels, and that the use of more sensory inputs reduces both training and test errors. To introduce the time-dimension into the learning and prediction process, previous sensory signal samples were used together with the current ones. An important feature for control was introduced: an early prediction of stimulation events, which provides a time interval during which the subject can be informed about coming stimulation. ALNs were tested in predicting the stimulation events up to two seconds in advance.

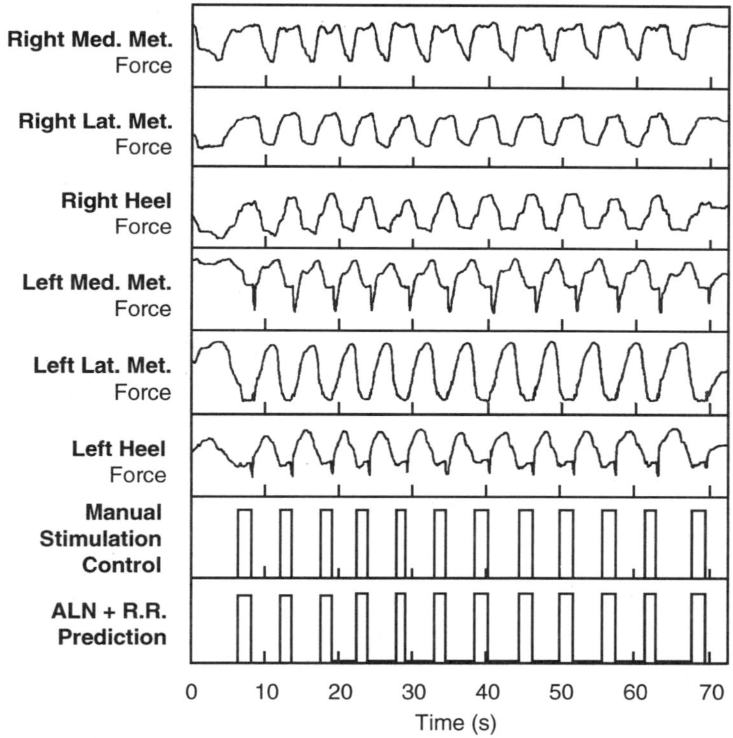

Figure 18.10. Signals of force sensors and manual stimulation during data capture. ALN +R. R. is the result of training shown upon replay. Excellent agreement must still be checked for generalization.

After the training, ALNs were tested on the data set used for ALN training. If their approximation of the output control signal did not contain any functional errors (extra or missing stimuli), they were tested on new data which were not used during the training. If there were no functional errors in predicted output control signals, a similar test was repeated, but this time during real-time manually controlled walking. The subject still controlled the stimulation manually, but this time she heard a buzzing noise from the controller interface every time the ALNs predicted the stimulation should be ON. The conditions of this test were the closest possible to those of ALN real-time control of the stimulation. After this test was passed without any functional errors, the next task was to apply the ALNs in real-time control of stimulation for FES-assisted walking. The subject, after standing up from the wheelchair, took one or more manually controlled steps and then the ALN control was switched ON and put in parallel with the manual control, which remained active as a functional override.

Results obtained so far demonstrate the capability of ALNs trained on manually controlled FES-assisted walking to generalize to automatically controlled FES-assisted walking. It was also demonstrated that the generalization is satisfactory not only over the same walking session, but also over several days or weeks (Kostov 1995). This result implies that, using this approach to design, a control system may be quite robust and frequent retrainings of the ALNs (calibration) may not be necessary. It remains to be seen how fast the walking pattern changes, requiring new ALN training or retraining of the existing ALNs. In the case that ALNs can generalize over long periods of time, an integrated control system (ICS) can be built consisting of two parts: an FES control fitting station and the FES controller itself. The FES controller can be miniaturized and built into a portable neuroprosthetic device. The control rules can be generated in the laboratory or at home using an FES control fitting station, which can be based on a small notebook computer with data acquisition extensions. After the control rules are produced, they can be downloaded to the portable FES controller, which can be used independently.

Inductive learning (IL) was also tested for control of FES (Kostov 1995). It was used to measure the relative importance of sensors: the sensory set was reduced from ten sensors to only four sensors of highest importance. IL was evaluated in a complex environment for cloning the control rules for walking of a subject with *complete* spinal cord injury. It was demonstrated that IL is also capable of cloning the skill of skilled subjects in controlling two-channel stimulation for FES-assisted walking. ALN and IL techniques were compared on a larger sample recorded from six subjects. It was demonstrated that, although IL generates its decision trees faster and with lower training error, the ALNs have better generalization. A practical implication of this result is that IL may be better suited for use in control systems where the training data set represents the domain very well. It is obvious that training sets acquired during walking of subjects with SCI cannot represent all possible situations, because some high-risk situations that would be of interest as a part of a training set could give rise to possible injuries (e.g. instability leading to a fall). Both techniques give better results if previous samples are used together with current ones. Also, both techniques are capable of predicting future stimulation events. Overall performance was better with ALNs than with IL, which was crucial for deciding which machine learning technique to use for the design of an integrated control system.

18.6. Conclusions

The primary target of this work was the design of an upper level controller for a neuroprosthetic device to control FES for walking in SCI patients. To prepare for automatic generation of control rules, manually controlled FES-assisted walking of subjects with incomplete spinal cord injury was studied. Manually controlled stimulation for walking is important in the rehabilitation of SCI subjects as it provides the subject with a complete, easy and reliable way to learn how the muscles react to different stimulation conditions. It also remains the backup control system for stimulation during the development of more sophisticated control systems. Various sensors were evaluated for use as a source of sensory feedback information. It was concluded that an affordable array of force sensors built into the subjects' shoe insoles can provide a reliable and reproducible source of feedback information for design of control rules.

Automatic control of walking using a rule-based system resulted in faster walking (a shorter gait cycle) and longer walking sessions. Although successful, this form of automatic control revealed the difficult problem of generating control rules, originating in the subjects' differing stimulation needs, walking skills and walking patterns. Hand-crafting rules for one person does not guarantee transferability to other patients. Machine learning techniques which can generate the control rules automatically were proposed as a solution to this problem.

ALNs were evaluated for cloning the manual skill of a skilled subject or therapist in controlling one channel of stimulation for FES-assisted walking. The capability of ALNs to generate control rules from manually controlled stimulation was demonstrated. The ALN was also successful in predicting stimulation events up to two seconds in advance.

After ALN training, the result was tested on the training set, on a data set not used in training, and in real-time walking, where stimuli were given by the patient and the ALN automatic stimulation was indicated by a buzzer. After these tests were passed without any functional errors, the ALN could be used in real-time control of stimulation for FES-assisted walking. The subject, after standing up from the wheelchair, took one or more manually controlled steps and then ALN control was switched ON and put in parallel with the manual control, which remained active as a functional override.

Results obtained so far demonstrate capability of ALNs trained on manually controlled FES-assisted walking to generalize to automatically control FES-assisted walking. It was also demonstrated that the generalization is satisfactory not only within the same walking session, but also can extend up to several days.

This result suggests that the controller resulting from ALN training may be quite robust, and that frequent retrainings of the ALN may not be necessary. It remains to be seen how fast the walking pattern changes in a way requiring new ALN training or further training of the existing ALN.

18.7. References

(Armstrong 1991) W. Armstrong, A. Dwelly, J.-D. Liang, D. Lin, S. Reynolds, "Learning and Generalization in Adaptive Logic Networks," in *Artificial Neural Networks, Proceedings of the 1991 International Conference on Artificial Neural Networks (ICANN'91)*, ed.s Kohonen, K. Makisara, O. Simula, J. Kangas (Elsevier Science Publishing Co. Inc., New York, 1991), vol. 2, pp. 1173-1176.

(Armstrong 1992) W.W. Armstrong and M.M. Thomas, Atree 2.7 ALN development system for Windows 3.x. Available from ftp.cs.ualberta.ca in pub/atree/atre27.exe with C++ source code and extensive on-line help.

(Armstrong 1993) W.W. Armstrong, R.B. Stein, A. Kostov, M. Thomas, P. Baudin, P. Gervais, D. Popovic, "Application of adaptive logic networks and dynamics to study and control of human movement," *Second Int'l Symp. on 3D Analysis of Human Movement* (Poitiers, June 30 - July 3, 1993), pp. 81-84.

(Armstrong 1994) W.W. Armstrong, M.M. Thomas, "Control of a vehicle active suspension system using adaptive logic networks," available as a compressed PostScript® file from ftp.cs.ualberta.ca in pub/atree/wcnnpub.ps.Z.

(Armstrong 1995) W.W. Armstrong, M.M. Thomas, Atree 3.0 ALN development system demonstration program for Windows 3.x. From ftp.cs.ualberta.ca in pub/atree/aln3demo.zip (binary mode).

(Hecht-Nielsen 1990) Robert Hecht-Nielsen, *Neurocomputing* (Addison-Wesley, 1990).

(Kostov 1992) Aleksandar Kostov, Richard B. Stein, William W. Armstrong, Monroe Thomas, "Evaluation of Adaptive Logic Networks for Control of Walking in Paralyzed Patients," *14th Ann. Int'l Conf. IEEE Engineering in Medicine and Biology Society* (Paris, France, Oct. 29 - Nov. 1, 1992), vol.4, pp. 1332-1334.

(Kostov 1994) Aleksandar Kostov, Richard B. Stein, Dejan Popovic, W.W. Armstrong, "Improved Methods for Control of FES for Locomotion," *Proc. International Federation of Automatic Control (IFAC) Symposium on Modeling and Control in Biomedical Systems* (Galveston, Texas, USA, March 27 - 30, 1994).

(Kostov 1995) Aleksandar Kostov, "Machine Learning Techniques for the Control of FES-assisted Locomotion after Spinal Cord Injury," *PhD Thesis*, (Department of Neuroscience, University of Alberta, Edmonton, Alberta, Canada, 1995).

(Miller 1991) W.T. Miller, III, Richard S. Sutton and Paul Werbos, *Neural Networks for Control* (MIT Press, Cambridge, MA, 1990).

(Popovic 1993) D.B. Popovic, R.B. Stein, K.L. Jovanovic, R. Dai, A. Kostov, W.W. Armstrong, "Sensory Nerve Recording for Closed-Loop Control to Restore Motor Functions," *IEEE Trans. Biomed. Eng.* **40** (1994) 1024 - 1031.

(Stein 1993) Richard B. Stein, Marc Belanger, Garry Wheeler, Marquerite Wieler, Dejan B. Popovic, Arthur Prochazka, Lyle A. Davis, "Electrical Systems for Improving Locomotion After Incomplete Spinal Cord Injury: An Assessment," *Arch. Phys. Med. Rehabil.* **74** (1993) 954 - 959.

(Supynuk 1992) Allen G. Supynuk, William W. Armstrong, "Adaptive Logic Networks and Robot Control," *Proc. Vision Interface Conference '92*, also called AI/VI/GI '92, (Vancouver, BC, May 11-15, 1992), pp. 181 - 186.

19. SYNTHESIZE, OPTIMIZE, ANALYZE, REPEAT (SOAR): APPLICATION OF NEURAL NETWORK TOOLS TO ECG PATIENT MONITORING†

RAYMOND WATROUS, GEOFFREY TOWELL, AND MARTIN S. GLASSMAN
Siemens Corporate Research, 755 College Road East
Princeton, New Jersey 08540, USA
E-mail: watrous@learning.scr.siemens.com

ABSTRACT

Results are reported from the application of tools for synthesizing, optimizing and analyzing neural networks to an ECG Patient Monitoring task. A neural network was synthesized from a rule-based classifier and optimized over a set of normal and abnormal heartbeats. The classification error rate on a separate and larger test set was reduced by a factor of 2. Sensitivity analysis of the synthesized and optimized networks revealed informative differences. Analysis of the weights and unit activations of the optimized network enabled a reduction in size of the network by a factor of 40% without loss of accuracy.

19.1. Introduction

It has been pointed out that learning in complex domains is intractable without sufficient domain knowledge.[1] Consequently, the instantiation of domain knowledge in neural network models used in learning is of considerable interest. Once instantiated in a neural network model, domain knowledge can be refined by methods of nonlinear numerical optimization using gradient descent. This optimization results in domain knowledge which has been refined in a statistically disciplined manner.

In this paper, we describe several tools for synthesizing, optimizing and analyzing neural networks and present some results of applying these tools to a signal processing and classification task. The task is to detect the presence of potentially life-threatening arrhythmias in an electrocardiogram (ECG) signal. Domain knowledge in the area of arrhythmia detection was provided by Siemens Medical Electronics (SME) in the form of rules which were designed to distinguish ventricular premature beats (VPBs) from normal beats.

---

†This paper appeared previously in the *Proceedings of the Third International Congress on Air- and Structure-Borne Sound and Vibration*, June 13-15, 1994, Montréal, Québéc, pp. 997-1004, and the *Proceedings of the 1993 Symposium on Nonlinear Theory and its Applications*, December 5-10, Honolulu, Hawaii, pp. 565-570.

19.2. Synthesis

It has been shown that a neural network can be synthesized from any set of Boolean clauses.[5-6] That is, the architecture, unit offsets and interconnection strengths of a neural network can be determined directly from a set of disjunctions, conjunctions and negations of binary-valued propositions. The network architecture derives from the syntax of the Boolean expressions and the weight values are constrained by the functional form of the network and the representation of TRUE/FALSE.

Given the binary-valued logic of Boolean clauses, a representation of TRUE/FALSE has to be chosen in implementing the corresponding neural network. Call V_T the representation of TRUE and V_F the representation of FALSE. Neural network units are generally chosen to be continuous valued functions with continuous derivatives so that optimization of the network by gradient descent can be carried out. Since the unit function selected for use in this neural network was the sigmoidal function, $y(x) = (1 + e^{-x})^{-1}$, which has values between 0 and 1, V_T and V_F were chosen to be symmetric about 0.5 and were parameterized by δ as $1 - \delta$ and δ respectively. Call C_T and C_F the input values of x for which the output is TRUE or FALSE, respectively; consequently, $C_T = \beta$ and $C_F = -\beta$, where $\beta = \ln(\frac{1-\delta}{\delta})$.

Happily, the set of rules comprising the SME arrhythmia detection portion of the ECG patient monitoring algorithm were easily translated into Boolean clauses. The Boolean clause formulation consisted of a single disjunction of 14 conjunctions of subsets of 24 propositions. These propositions were defined with respect to a set of 8 waveshape and timing features derived from the QRS complex extracted from the ECG signal.

19.2.1. Propositions

In the case of the SME classifier, the propositions were expressed as relational operators applied to a single integer-valued feature with respect to a critical value. Since most propositions were expressed using the relational operators that include equality ($\leq$ and $\geq$), the proposition was clearly TRUE when the input was at the critical value; that is, C_T. However, it was still necessary to determine the input value C_F for which the proposition became false. Since the critical values varied over several orders of magnitude, it was decided to have the proposition become false if the input fell short of the critical value by a fixed percentage rather than by a fixed amount. Those propositions which were expressed *without* equality were modified to include equality, based on the fact that the input features are integer valued.

Once the input values for which the proposition became true (C_T) or false (C_F) were established, the neural network instantiation was straightforward. For each proposition, a unit was synthesized with a weight $\omega = \frac{2\beta}{C_T - C_F}$ and an offset $\theta = -\beta(\frac{C_T + C_F}{C_T - C_F})$.

19.2.2. Clauses

The synthesis of a network from Boolean clauses is simplified if the clauses are expressed in disjunctive or conjunctive normal form. For each disjunction/conjunction, a single unit is synthesized with the link weights and offset chosen so that the output of the unit has the value V_T only when the corresponding logical relation is TRUE.

For the case of conjunction, assume there are *n positive* antecedents (i.e., antecedents which must be true) and *m negative* antecedents (i.e., antecedents which must be false). Assume that the conjunction is instantiated as a single unit with weights ω^+ from the positive antecedents and weights ω^- from the negative antecedents. Recall that the propositions take on the values V_T or V_F according as they are TRUE or FALSE.

The conjunction requires that:

$$n\omega^+ V_T + m\omega^- V_F + \theta = \beta \tag{19.1}$$

whereas if a single positive antecedent is false, or a single negative antecedent is true, the conjunction is false. Solving these constraints leads to the following values:

$$\omega^+ = \frac{2\beta}{1 - 2\delta} \tag{19.2}$$

with $\omega^- = -\omega^+$ and

$$\theta = \beta - \omega^+(n - (m+n)\delta) \tag{19.3}$$

For the disjunctive case, the relation is FALSE only if all its antecedents are false, whereas if a single positive antecedent is true, or a single negative antecedent is false, the disjunction is true. These constraints are again satisfied by $\omega^+ = \frac{2\beta}{1-2\delta}$ and $\omega^- = -\omega^+$, while

$$\theta = -\beta + \omega^+(m - (m+n)\delta) \tag{19.4}$$

19.2.3. Instantiation of SME Classifier

A neural network instantiation of the SME classifier was synthesized with propositions satisfying the condition that a relative difference of 1% in the input at the critical value caused the proposition to change from TRUE to FALSE. The resulting network, depicted in Figure 19.1, yielded identical performance to the original set of rules.

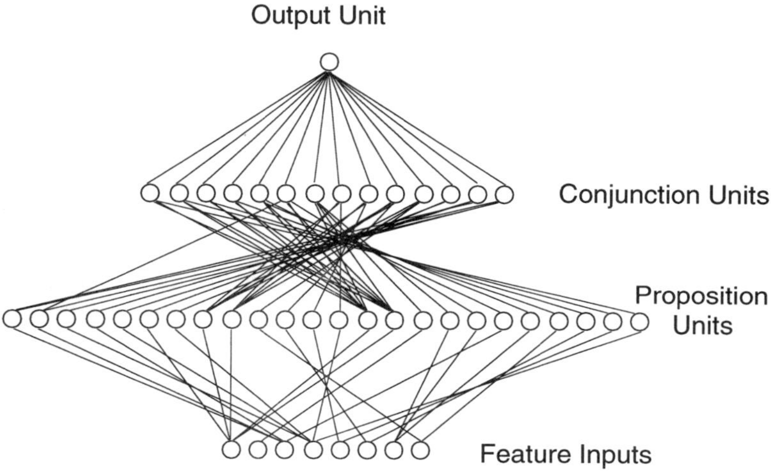

Figure 19.1. Neural Network Instantiation of the SME Classifier.

19.3. Optimization

The gradient of the output of a neural network with respect to the parameters of the network can be efficiently computed.[4] Consequently, the network can be optimized by standard nonlinear methods of gradient descent.

For the ECG application, there are several large data bases available, including the MIT/BIH database, which contains approximately 100,000 heartbeats that have been labeled by expert cardiologists. A subset of this data base was used for training purposes and the remainder for testing.

It has been shown that minimization of the mean squared error (MSE) leads to an estimate of the posterior probability of the class given the input.[3] This measure includes the *prior* probability of the class, which is assumed to be represented in the distribution of the training samples. Since examples of arrhythmias are relatively rare in the standard ECG data bases, the prior probability of a normal beat is quite high. However, since the cost of misclassifying an abnormal beat as normal is high, this cost should be reflected in the function being minimized in training. Alternatively, the data used for training can be filtered to balance the distribution of normal/abnormal beats to effectively increase the prior probability of an abnormal beat.

Consequently, a clustering algorithm was used to select beats that were maximally distinct according to a standard distance metric. In selecting maximally distinct examples, the clustering algorithm focused attention on what might be considered prototypical rather than frequent instances. The clustering algorithm nearly equalized the number of normal and abnormal beats, which increased the effective prior probability of an abnormal beat and the effective cost of misclassifying an abnormal beat. Clustering also had the advantage of reducing the number of training samples by a factor of 50.

A neural network synthesized from the SME rule set was optimized on selected heartbeats from 20 patients chosen from the MIT/BIH data base by minimizing the mean squared error between the classifications given by the network and the correct classifications. The performance of the optimized network was compared with that of the original rule base on these patients and it was found that the classification error rate had been reduced by a factor of 2. A similar improvement in performance was obtained on the remainder of the MIT/BIH data base. The error rate was reduced on two other standard data bases by factors of 4 and 5.

19.4. Analysis

19.4.1. Sensitivity Analysis

Having instantiated the SME classifier in the form of a differentiable neural network, it became possible to compute the sensitivity of the classifier output to its input features.

Following a method introduced by Kuhn,[2] the sensitivities were ordered by the value of the output unit; this allowed the sensitivities to be interpreted with respect to the correctness of the classifier. Shown in the upper panel of Figure 19.2 are the sensitivities of the output of the SME classifier to input features for normal beats, sorted from left to right by increasing correctness of the response.

Note that sensitivity is near zero, as represented by a medium gray level, for most features across most templates; there are only a few darker and lighter regions corresponding to positive and negative sensitivities, respectively. These regions are sporadic both in their relationship to the output of the classifier and in their values which occasionally alternate between black and white. For the most part, the regions of nonzero sensitivity occur when the classification decision is fairly stable. This suggests that *fine tuning the features may have little effect on the performance of the classifier*. This is important because improvements to individual features which are pursued on the basis of their role in a few classification errors may not have the desired effect of overall performance, because the classification is decided on the basis of other features.

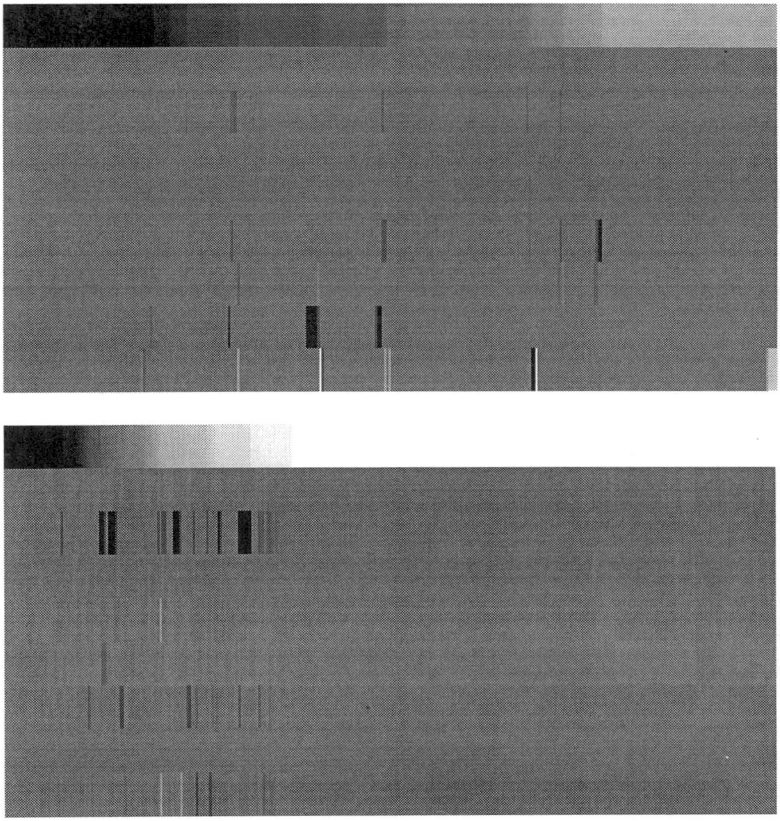

Figure 19.2. Sensitivity of SME Classifier to Input Features of Normal Templates. The inputs are ordered from left to right by the activation of the output of the classifier, which is shown in the upper swath, from less correct to more correct. Zero sensitivity is shown as a medium gray level with positive sensitivities increasingly black and negative sensitivities increasingly white. The upper panel shows the sensitivities of the original classifier and the lower panel shows the sensitivities of the optimized classifier.

The sensitivities of the *optimized* neural network classifier are shown in the lower panel of Figure 19.2. Note that the nonzero sensitivities are now concentrated in the region of transition between correct and incorrect classification. Generally, the sensitivities are near zero in the regions where the classifier is definitely correct or definitely incorrect. Furthermore, there is a high positive sensitivity to a certain feature which is not balanced by a negative sensitivity for other tokens. This was considered unusual and suggested a possibly erratic feature; this possibility was later confirmed by SME.

19.4.2. Network Interpretation

Analysis of the optimized network revealed that the critical values for the proposition units had changed by different amounts for different propositions. It was also found that the steepness of transition from TRUE to FALSE was essentially unchanged. This suggested the proposition units might be convertible back into binary rules with new threshold values.

The weighted contribution of each feature and antecedent to each conjunctive or disjunctive unit was also analyzed, working backward from the output unit. Units which contributed a constant (or zero) amount were replaced by adding the same constant value to the unit offset. By an analysis of this kind, 6 conjunction units were identified that could be replaced by constant values. When these conjunction units were removed from the network, an additional 8 propositions became unnecessary and were also removed. This reduced the network from 39 to 24 units and from 121 to 76 links. When tested on the training set and the test set, the reduced network yielded identical performance. Thus, an optimized network, reduced in size by 40%, maintained an increase in performance over the unoptimized network of a factor of 2.

19.5. Conclusions

We concluded from our experience that the instantiation of a set of hand-tuned rules in a differentiable nonlinear model:

1. Permits the disciplined acquisition of a refined model which represents a statistically validated theory, when combined with numerical optimization over a large data base.
2. Provides a means for evaluating the utility of the input data, when combined with sensitivity analysis.
3. Makes it possible to simplify the optimized network by deleting extraneous units, when combined with other analysis tools.
4. May also enable optimization of the features extracted from the original signal, if they can be similarly expressed in a differentiable form.

We also concluded that these tools are likely to be applicable to a very large number of signal processing and classification systems, whether medical, automotive, or industrial.

19.6. Acknowledgments

We are glad to acknowledge the support of Siemens Medical Electronics and, in particular, the contributions of Peter Martin, Steve Marinello and Bill Murray. We also acknowledge the constructive participation of Dr. Gary M. Kuhn, Siemens Corporate Research.

19.7. References

1. S. Geman, E. Bienenstock and R. Doursat, "Neural networks and the bias/variance dilemma," *Neural Computation* **4** (1992) 1-58.
2. G. Kuhn, "Joint optimization of classifier and feature space in speech recognition," in *Proceedings of the International Joint Conference on Neural Networks* (IEEE, Piscataway, NJ, 1992), vol. 4, pp. 709-714.
3. J. Makhoul, "Pattern recognition properties of neural networks," in *Neural Networks for Signal Processing: Proceedings of the 1991 IEEE Workshop*, ed.s B.H. Juang, S.Y. Kung and C.A. Kamm (IEEE Signal Processing Society, 1991), pp. 173-187.
4. D.E. Rumelhart, G. Hinton and R. Williams, "Learning internal representations by error propagation," in *Parallel Distributed Processing: Explorations in the Microstructure of Cognition: Volume I Foundation*, ed.s D.E. Rumelhart, J.L. McClelland and the PDP research group (MIT Press, Cambridge, MA, 1986), chapter 8.
5. G.G. Towell, J.W. Shavlik and M.O Noordewier, "Refinement of approximately correct domain theories by knowledge-based neural networks," in *Proceedings of the Eighth National Conference on Artificial Intelligence* (AAAI Press, Boston, MA, 1990), pp. 861-866.
6. R.L. Watrous, *Speech Recognition using Connectionist Network*, PhD thesis, (University of Pennsylvania, 1988).

20. DIAGNOSTIC SYSTEM FOR DETECTION AND ANALYSIS OF AUDITORY EVOKED POTENTIALS

YURI V. ORLOV, I.G. PERSIANTSEV, S.P. REBRIK, A.A. DEVIATOV, JU.S. SHUGAI
Microelectronics Department, Nuclear Physics Institute, Moscow State University
Moscow 119899, Russia
E-mail: orlov@neuro.npi.msu.su

and

A.V. KURGANSKIJ
Psychological Department, Moscow State University
Moscow 119899, Russia

ABSTRACT

The diagnostic system using artificial neural nets (ANN) for an objective hearing loss examination of humans by the auditory evoked potentials (EP) method, has been developed and tested.

20.1. Introduction

Auditory evoked potentials (AEPs) are electric signals of the brain that appear in the response to auditory stimulus. Most widely used AEPs are short-latency brainstem auditory response (BAER) and long-latency cortex AEP, that are often called long-latency response (LLR).

For BAER acquisition, a very short (about 0.1 ms) and consequently broad-band auditory signal is used. This means that the results of a patient examination based on BAER are frequency-insensitive and cannot be used to determine degree of hearing loss at specific frequencies. BAERs are reliably detected at 1-2 months-old children, and can be used for hard-of-hearing detection at early ages.

For LLR acquisition, a relatively long (about 40 ms) tone burst is used. This provides a possibility to determine hearing loss versus frequency and to use this dependency for hearing correction with the help of hearing aids. LLR are reliably detected at 1-2 years-old children.

As all EPs are registered by the signal accumulation method, in the process of examination one should provide for reliable level of EP averaging at which the resulting waveform becomes stable and have no tendency to change with further accumulations. For BAER and for LLR signals typical number of accumulation cycles is about 1000-2000 and 40-50 respectively.

Using of BAER and LLR make it possible to detect hard-of-hearing problems at early ages and to help in the hearing aids fitting for children. AEP audiometry having a high diagnosis value is at the same time a laborious process for a physician and a tiresome procedure for a patient. High qualification required from an expert interpreting EP waveforms, precludes to some extent from wide EP introduction into clinical practice. Significant duration of the procedure (40-50 min) is also a serious obstacle on the way to wide method's application for screening purposes.

20.2. Data Collection

EP recording was performed at the otorhinolaryngology department of The First Moscow child's hospital. Basic characteristics of the audiometer used correspond to those of traditional computer audiometers.

Over 60 children aging from 2 months to 15 years were examined. The main part of the patients (80%) had normal hearing, the remaining part had hard-of-hearing problems of different nature. Before AEP testing the hearing function was examined by the pure-tone threshold audiometry (for children older than 5 years) and/or by acoustic impedance measurement method. A number of children were sent for examination from the neurology department for brainstem testing.

BAER and LLR registration was conducted in strict accordance with traditional protocols. LLR records were taken at tone burst frequency of 1000 Hz.

The system of data acquisition provided comprehensive way of data recording: for LLR records the result of 30 accumulation cycles together with 30 single records were stored, and for BAER records sum of 2000 accumulations together with 10 records of 200 accumulations each, were stored. This data structure provided for development of a new system that was aimed at less accumulations than traditional, it also provided for possibility of real-time-recording simulation for testing of the system.

20.3. ANN-Based Filter

One of the objectives of current research was implementation of some kind of waveform preprocessing that could make detection and interpretation easier for an expert and make this procedure possible at as low accumulation number as possible. For this purpose it was suggested to use an ANN-based filter.[1,2] The filter enhances clinically important EP peaks and suppresses random spikes that have no relation to brain response on periodic stimulation.

ANN filter processes a record that is the result of some number of accumulations (starting with one accumulation and up to the full number prescribed by the protocol). ANN output is interpreted as a filtered out input record.

We used a feed forward multilayer neural network.[3] In all experiments with ANNs input and output layers had the same dimension. Number of neurons in the hidden layer was varied in 4-32 limits. After a series of additional experiments we have chosen an ANN with 250 neurons in the input and in the output layers and 16 neurons in the hidden layer. Hyperbolic tangent was taken as a transfer function of the hidden layer, and for the output layer a linear function was used.

ANN filter was trained by error back propagation method.[4] In the training procedure the next strategy was used. At the first stage the curves with maximal number of accumulations (2000 for BAER and 30 for LLR) were presented to the ANN. The same curves were used as the target outputs for the net. After reaching of a prescribed error level the task was complicated: ANN was supplied with curves with less accumulation number (e.g. 1000 for BAER and 15 for LLR), while target output was kept the same. In this way the ANN was taught to make a prognosis of the waveform corresponding to a large accumulation number knowing only a curve with small number of accumulations. In the training process the number of accumulations in the input curves was gradually reduced until the net was still capable to keep the error level on the desired level. Minimal accumulation number at which the net was still able to make a satisfactory prognosis was 200 for BAER and 3-5 for LLR. We should note that the limit of 200 accumulations was the result of existing data structure (we could not test lower values).

20.4. BAER Filter

According to the protocol, BAER registration requires 2000 accumulations for reaching of sufficient signal to noise ratio. This value depends on the degree to which stimulation exceeds the subject's hearing level. For normally hearing person 1000 accumulations are enough at 80-90 dB level, while at 30-40 dB level, which is close to the threshold, all 2000 accumulations are needed.

ANN filter for BAER extraction was trained at the set of 171 waveforms corresponding to different patients and different stimulation levels. Testing set consisted of 67 waveforms.

Comparison of the waveforms with 200 accumulations processed by the net and raw waveforms with 2000 accumulations showed that the net successfully performs the following transformations: 1) improves total signal to noise ratio; 2) restores peaks I-V, if they have been masked off by the noise at low accumulation number, but they are present at fully accumulated record; 3) swaps off positive and negative spikes that have no relation to the BAER.

One of the most advantageous features of the ANN filter is its processing of the I, III, and V peaks. Dependency of their latencies on stimulus intensity is one of the most important diagnosis factors of BAER method. The filter represents form and position of these peaks with good accuracy, despite the fact that position changes significantly with stimulation level. The other valuable feature of the ANN filter is that it has no tendency to show BAER peaks, when they are absent in the raw curve.

Preliminary estimations show that for normally hearing patients ANN filter preprocessing will provide reduction of the accumulation number from 1000 to 200 at 80-90 dB level and from 2000 to 600 at near threshold intensities (20-40 dB). This means reduction of the examination time by a factor of 5.

20.5. LLR Filter

According to the protocol, LLR registration requires up to 50 accumulations for reaching of sufficient signal to noise ratio. For normally hearing person 15 accumulations may be enough at 80-90 dB level, while at 0-10 dB level, which is close to the hearing threshold, 30-50 accumulations are needed.

ANN filter for LLR extraction was trained similarly to the case of BAER filter.

For the testing of the ANN filter performance human expert was asked to find out the absolute hearing thresholds for 29 subjects. Expert used either (1) standard EEG records, or (2) the same records processed by ANN filter prior to the visual presentation to the expert.

The results of comparison of expert's evaluation with and without using of ANN filter show that the use of ANN filter can allow to estimate the presence or absence of EP automatically at earlier stages (e.g. at 3-5 accumulations).

20.6. Hearing Threshold Determination Using BAER

An ANN system for hearing threshold determination on the basis of BAER[2] was trained on the data marked by a human expert.

The curves are recorded for different intensities of sound stimulus. The maximum number of curves in the set is 8. In practice the actual number of recorded curves may be smaller. During pattern presentation recorded curves are grouped together, while absent curves are substituted by zeroes. All 8 curves are presented simultaneously to the network input.

The output layer consists of 8 neurons also, by one neuron for each waveform in the input pattern. The ANN output represents a confidence of V peak detection for each curve. The value of hearing threshold is determined as that stimulus intensity when activity of output neurons begin to exceed the value of empirically chosen decision function.

The values of hearing thresholds determined for 2000 accumulation cycles and for 200 ones are the same, i.e. the significant decrease of the signal-to-noise ratio does not influence practically on the final evaluation of the hearing threshold.

20.7. Hearing Threshold Determination Using LLR

Hearing threshold determination using LLR is based on the measurement of LLR amplitude.

First experiments were done on the synthesized records. Background EEG was modeled on the basis of its typical Fourier spectrum. LLR form was approximated by analytical dependency of the form: $At^2exp(-t)$ with corresponding coefficients. In the case of synthesized waveforms signal amplitude is known with absolute accuracy, and its value can be used for training of the net. For EP amplitude estimation we used an ANN with one hidden layer having hyperbolic tangent transfer function and with one output neuron having linear transfer function.

Next, this approach was tested on more realistic waveforms. Real background EEG were mixed with the LLR-approximating function given above. This variant of training data gave close results to fully synthesized waveforms.

The ANN was tested on real LLR records taken at different stimulation intensities. The net was determining LLR amplitude and the resulting dependency of determined amplitude on stimulus intensity was further approximated by the function of the form: $A/(1+exp(B\ (x-C))$, where x stands for the stimulus intensity in dB, parameter B was fixed at 10 dB level, C and A parameters were adjusted by least squares procedure.

Assuming that dependency of LLR amplitude on the stimulus level is described by the above relation, one can interpret C parameter as the threshold value.

20.8. Conclusion

The above diagnostic system was tested on the clinical database and turned out to be promising. Also implementation of automatic procedure of patient examination was shown to be possible.

The developed approach allows one

- to detect clinically significant peaks;
- to suppress random spikes that are not related to evoked potentials;
- to measure amplitude of the peaks;
- to estimate the hearing threshold;
- to significantly reduce required number of data accumulation and consequently to reduce overall examination time;
- to reduce requirements for qualification of medical personnel interpreting examination results.

The developed approach may be used for brain monitoring either during surgical operation or for active determination of the drug dose required for a particular patient, and it may be also applied to other types of EPs and event-related responses.

The suggested methods of automatic hearing threshold detection make it possible to implement an adaptive procedure of patient examination. Namely, it is possible to scan the stimulus intensity range with a small number of accumulations, determining hearing threshold value roughly. Afterwards, the region of the threshold location can be examined more thoroughly with higher accumulation number.

20.9. References

1. Ya.M. Sapognikov, M.R. Bogomilsky, I.G. Persiantsev, *et. al.*, "Expert system for extraction of the evoked potentials," *International Symposium on the Modern Problem of Hearing Physiology and Pathology* (Moscow, Russia, 1993), pp. 39-40.
2. A.A. Deviatov, Yu.V. Orlov, I.G. Persiantsev, *et. al.*, "Application of Neural Nets for Acquisition And Processing of Auditory Evoked Potentials," in *Report on the First World Congress on Computation Medicine and Biology* (Austin, Texas, 1994).
3. R.P. Lippman, "An Introduction to Computing with Neural Nets," *IEEE ASSP Magazine* (1987) 4-22.
4. D.E. Rumelhart, G.E. Hinton and R.J. Williams, *Parallel Distributed Processing, Explorations in the Microstructures of Cognition, 1:Foundations* (MIT Press, Cambridge, MA, 1987), pp. 318-362.

21. DIAGNOSING CORONARY ARTERY DISEASE WITH A BACKPROPAGATION NEURAL NETWORK: LESSONS LEARNED

DAVID D. TURNER
Pacific Northwest National Laboratory†*, P.O. Box 999, MS K7-28*
Richland, Washington 99352, USA
E-mail: dd_turner@pnl.gov

and

EDWIN R. HOLMES, III, M.D.
Sacred Heart Medical Center, West 101 8th Avenue, TAF-C9
Spokane, Washington 99220, USA

ABSTRACT

The SPECT (single photon emitted computed tomography) procedure, while widely used for diagnosing coronary artery disease, is not a perfect technology. We have investigated using a backpropagation neural network to diagnose patients suffering from coronary artery disease that is independent from the SPECT procedure.

The raw thallium-201 scintigrams produced before the SPECT tomographic reconstruction were used as input patterns for the backpropagation neural network, and the diagnoses resulting mainly from cardiac catheterization as the desired outputs for each pattern. Several preprocessing techniques were applied to the scintigrams, in an attempt to improve the information to noise ratio. After using a procedure that extracted a subimage containing the heart from each scintigram, we used a data reduction technique, thereby encoding the scintigram in 12 values, which were the inputs to the backpropagation neural network.

The network was then trained. This network performed superbly for patients suffering from inferolateral disease (classifying 10 out of 10 correctly), but performance was less than optimal for cases involving other coronary zones.

While the scope of this project was limited to diagnosing coronary artery disease, this initial work can be extended to other medical imaging procedures, such as diagnosing breast cancer from a mammogram and evaluating lung perfusion studies.

21.1. Introduction

Coronary artery disease (CAD) is one of the leading causes of death for adults in the United States today. As the medical community proceeds to adopt new methodologies and techniques utilizing the power and versatility of computers, computer

---

†Pacific Northwest National Laboratory is a multiprogram national laboratory operated by Battelle Memorial Institute for the U.S. Department of Energy under Contract DE-AC06-76RLO 1830.

based diagnostic tools will become more important. Neural networks make up a class of these tools, but because of their ability to solve complex problems for which algebraic solution do not exist or are too complicated to be found, such as pattern recognition problems, they have a definite advantage over other technologies.

21.2. Current Technology

Today's current technology to aid in the diagnosis of CAD is the Single Photon Emission Computed Tomography procedure, or SPECT. While this is the most widely accepted tool in the United States for diagnosing CAD, it is far from perfect, resulting in many misdiagnoses.

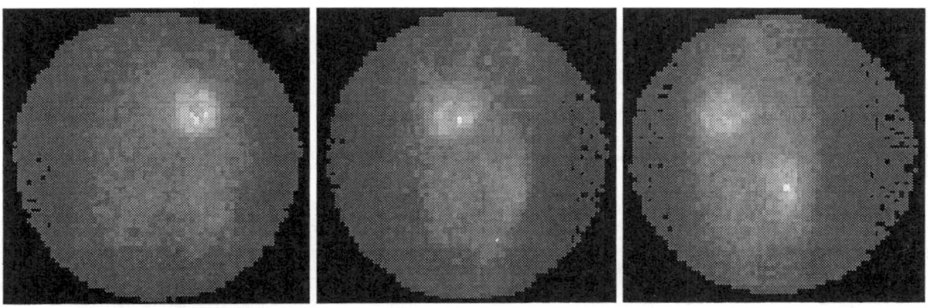

Figure 21.1. Examples of scintigrams produced by a gamma camera. These images are, from left to right, the anterior view, the 45° left anterior oblique view, and 70° left anterior oblique view.

When a patient is suspected of suffering from CAD after an interview with his or her doctor, the patient is subjected to the SPECT procedure. First, the patient is exercised to increase his or her heart rate to close to maximum. After this is reached, or it is no longer safe for the patient to exercise, the patient is injected with thallium 201, a radioactive isotope with a relatively short half life. This isotope is carried by the racing blood to the tissues of the heart. Soon after the patient's breathing rate returns to normal, a series of 32 planar images is taken of the patient's aid chest, from 45 degrees right anterior oblique to 45 degrees left posterior oblique, with a gamma camera. The time for each image is approximately 30-40 seconds. The camera is equipped with a low energy collimator and records the number of photons that are emitted from the patient's chest during each imaging time. After the images are completed, a computer algorithm backprojects these images to create a three dimensional model of the heart, and then a physician or technologist identifies one of the major axes of the heart in the model. The model is then sliced up along the principal axes, and the slices are used to create a "Bull's-eye plot." A Bull's-eye plot is a two dimensional polar graph where different regions of the graph correspond to specific walls of the heart, and the color of each section signifies the amount of thallium that is present in that wall of the heart. The more thallium there is, the better the blood flow to that spot. The physician then uses the Bull's-eye to identify areas that have little thallium, and therefore are not receiving the proper amount of blood; this indicates coronary artery disease in the artery that feeds that area of the heart.

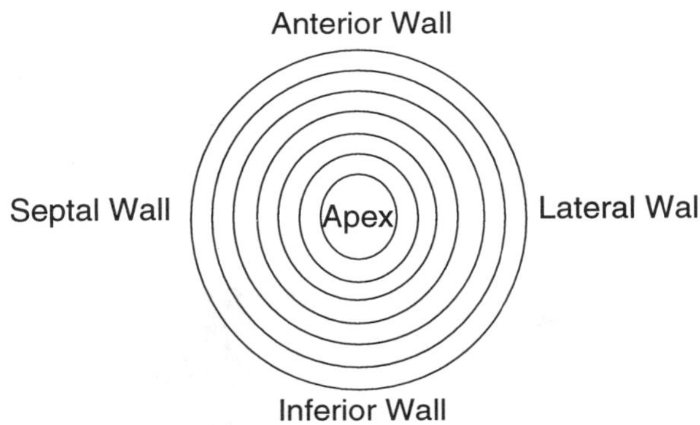

Figure 21.2. The Bull's-eye Plot. A two dimensional representation of the areas of the heart.

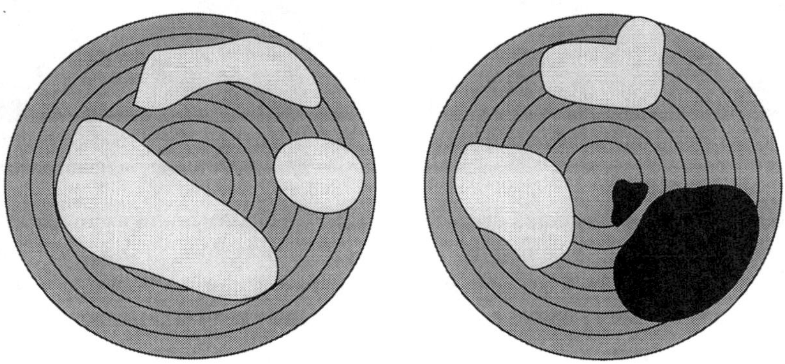

Figure 21.3. Examples of Bull's-eye plots. The plot on the left is that of a healthy patient, while the one on the right indicates CAD in the inferolateral wall.

However, as stated above, the SPECT procedure is not perfect. First, given the long amount of time needed for imaging the patient (close to 30 minutes, given the actual imaging time and the time needed for the camera to rotate to new positions), it is hard for many patients to remain motionless. If the patient moves during the imaging sequence, the reconstruction algorithm produces a faulty model of the heart, which leads to an erroneous bull's-eye and misdiagnoses. Another limitation of the SPECT is exposed if the physician or technologist incorrectly selects a line through the model that is not in actuality one of the principal axes. This again leads to misdiagnoses.

21.3. Using an Artificial Neural Network to Aid in Diagnosis of CAD

Our objective was to assess the feasibility and create a technology based on an artificial neural network that would aid in the detection and the diagnosis of CAD. We wanted to avoid as many of the pitfalls of the SPECT procedure as possible, so we decided to use the raw planar thallium scintigrams as the inputs to our technology.

Our approach was straightforward. The raw scintigrams are inherently noisy, and therefore we desired some preprocessing techniques that would reduce the data and enhance the information to noise ratio. We decided to use backpropagation neural networks as the core of our technology, because of their simplicity and the fact that they have a supervised learning scheme. Our initial goal was simple: we wanted to distinguish between two cases, either the patient suffered from coronary artery disease or was healthy.

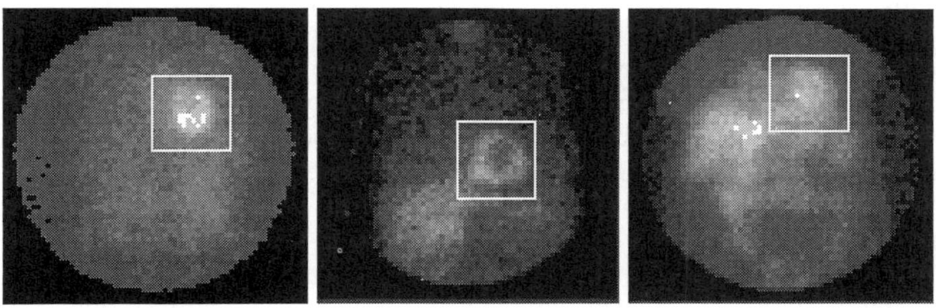

Figure 21.4. Examples of the subimages that were extracted from the original images. Notice the amount of irrelevant data that is removed.

Our first step was to reduce the data. Each scintigram is a 64x64 pixel image, but the heart was less than 10% of this image. Therefore, we created a simple expert system to examine each image and extract a 19x19 pixel subimage that contained the heart. Not only did this reduce the amount of data for each patient, it also removed such organs as the liver and most of the lungs, which also attracts thallium and could possibly cause confusion for the neural network.

Alas, at the time of this work, the number of patients for which we had both data and diagnoses was small (54 patients). Therefore, if we chose to use the entire 19x19 image as an input to the network, the degrees of freedom would have been extremely large. We needed to reduce the subimages further. We decided to "sectorize" each of the subimages into 12 sectors, then we averaged a value for each of the sectors. In this way, we reduced each scintigram to 12 values, which along with the image number were to be the inputs to our network.

We used a three layer feedforward network, with 13 input nodes, 5 hidden nodes, and one output node. We trained on a set of 31 patients, 15 of which suffered from coronary artery disease. The training was stopped when the error on the validation set, which consisted of 10 patients, five of which were diseased, inflected.

The network was then used to diagnose the patients in the data sets. Of the patients in the training set, 14 of the 16 healthy patients and 14 of the 15 diseased patients were diagnosed correctly. The patients in the validation set were all correctly diagnosed. Since these sets of patients are used to train the network, they are not true indicators of the performance of the network. Therefore, another disjoint set of patients was diagnosed by the network. Of the 7 diseased patients, 4 were diagnosed correctly, while 4 of the 6 healthy patients were diagnosed correctly.

We proceeded to analyze why the network did not perform as well for the independent testing set as for the other sets. By looking at the distribution of the CAD for the patients in the diseased sets, it was noticed that all of the diseased patients in both the testing and validation sets suffered from CAD in the inferolateral wall of the heart. However, only 4 of the 7 diseased patients in the independent testing set had inferolateral disease; the other three had CAD in other coronary zones. Furthermore, the diseased patients that were misclassified by the network were the 3 patients suffering from CAD in coronary zones other than the inferolateral region.

21.4. Conclusions

Our network was able to distinguish between patients that suffered from coronary artery disease in the inferolateral wall of the heart form those who didn't. Therefore, we feel that we have met our objective, and have demonstrated that it is feasible to use an artificial network technology to aid in the diagnosis of CAD. By utilizing a larger database of patients, with care taken so that all of the coronary zones are well represented, a neural network can be expected to perform very well. Also, the data reduction process helped to reduce the degrees of freedom in the network, but experimentation may discover a better process that not only reduces the amount of data but also helps to enhance in the information within the scintigram.

22. COMPRESSION AND MODEL REDUCTION: A CASE STUDY

THOMAS LOFARO
Department of Pure and Applied Mathematics, Washington State University
Pullman, Washington 99163-3113, USA
E-mail: lofaro@delta.math.wsu.edu

and

NANCY KOPELL
Department of Mathematics, Boston University
Boston, Massachusetts 02215, USA

ABSTRACT

We discuss a method by which the dynamics of a network of coupled neurons can be captured in a one-dimensional map. The network used as an example of this technique consists of a pair of neurons, one of which is an endogenous burster and the other excitable, but not bursting in the absence of phasic input. The reduction is accomplished by decomposing the flow into fast and slow subsystems, each operating on a distinct time scale. A "map of knees" is constructed using singular perturbation techniques. A concise expression for this map is developed by introducing time coordinates to each stable branch of the slow manifold. The compression associated with the fast subsystem is used to determine the qualitative properties of the map.

22.1. Introduction

In this paper we illustrate, by way of example, a method to capture the dynamics of a network of voltage-gated conductance equations in a low-dimensional map. This technique utilizes ideas from geometric singular perturbation theory to decompose the flow into two subsystems, each operating on a different timescale. The so-called "slow system" consists of flows on stable branches of the slow manifold and the "fast-system" is a network of "jumps" between these branches. This leads to the construction of a Poincaré-like map which we refer to as a "map of knees." A simple expression for the derivative of this map is obtained by introducing time coordinates onto each stable branch of the slow manifold. This allows for a straightforward analysis of the dynamics of the map of knees and hence the dynamics of the original model as well.

We begin with a brief introduction of the model used to illustrate these techniques. In Reference 3 we discuss the behavior of a network consisting of two

---

†This research was supported in part by the U.S. National Institute of Mental Health (NIMH) under grant MH47150

model neurons that are coupled via reciprocal inhibition. One of the model neurons is an endogenous burster (denoted PD) and the other is excitable, but not bursting in the absence of phasic input (denoted LP). The primary component in the model of each of these neurons is the nondimensional Morris-Lecar equations.[6]

$$\begin{aligned} \dot{v} &= I + g_k w(v_k - v) + g_\ell (v_\ell - v) + g_{ca} m_\infty(v)(1-v) \\ \dot{w} &= \varepsilon \lambda(v)(w_\infty(v) - w) \end{aligned} \tag{22.1}$$

An additional differential equation describing a hyperpolarizing inward current, I_h, is included in the description of the LP neuron. For a more complete description of these equations and the resulting model see Reference 3. In order to illustrate the methods used to analyze these models, we will ignore the role of I_h in this paper. The resulting model then consists of two copies of Eq. (22.1) coupled together by terms modeling mutual inhibition.

We account for the different uncoupled behaviors of the LP and PD by choosing different values of the parameter I in each pair of equations. Depending on the choice of this parameter, Equations (22.1) have either a unique asymptotically stable critical point or an asymptotically stable limit cycle. The system describing the LP (v_1, w_1 coordinates) will exhibit the former of these two possibilities, while the system describing the PD (v_2, w_2 coordinates) will have the latter.

We assume that the coupling between the two neurons is Heaviside (i.e. either on or off) and that the effect of inhibitory coupling is that if neuron i is firing then the v_j-nullcline of neuron j is lowered by some fixed amount depending only on v_j.

22.2. Model Analysis

A primary tool in the analysis of this model is geometric singular perturbation theory, a technique which can be used if we assume the parameter ε in Eq. (22.1) is small. In the limiting case $\varepsilon = 0$ there are two distinct subsystems. The "fast system" is obtained by setting $\varepsilon = 0$ directly. This gives a curve of critical points found by setting the right hand side of the $\dot{v}$ equation equal to 0. This curve, known as the v-nullcline, is cubic shaped with the left and right branches of this curve being asymptotically stable critical points for the fast system. In essence, the variable$w$ acts as a parameter for the fast system. The "slow system" is obtained by multiplying the left hand sides of Eq. (22.1) by ε and canceling where appropriate. Upon setting $\varepsilon = 0$, trajectories of the slow system lie on v-nullcline and satisfy the $\dot{w}$ differential equation. Because solutions of the slow system exist on this curve, it is often referred to as a slow manifold.

We can construct a singular solution by "gluing" together pieces of the fast and slow system in the natural way, with transitions between the two systems occurring at the extrema (or knees) of the v-nullcline. Theorems of Mischenko and Rosov,[5] and Bonet[1] guarantee that in most instances for $\varepsilon \ll 1$, periodic solutions constructed in this manner correspond to solutions of the original differential equations. Given a knee K we can define a first return map h in the usual manner. Since the dimension of a knee is 1 less than the dimension of the slow manifold and the slow manifold is at least 1 dimension smaller than the phase space, h is a function acting on a submanifold of at least 2 dimensions less than the original phase space.

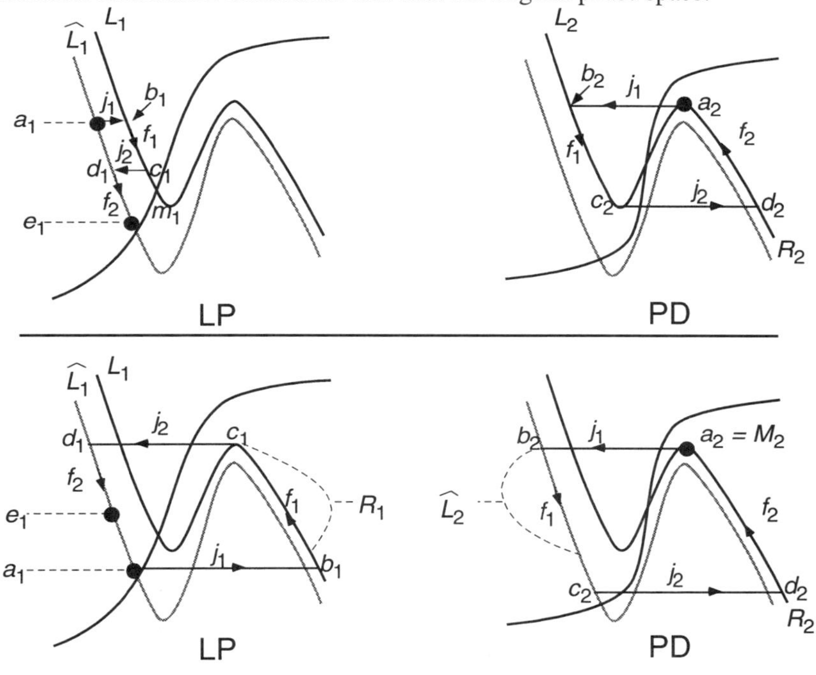

Figure 22.1. **Top:** A graphical representation of h_1. The initial condition is the point $p = (a_1, a_2)$ and $h_1(p) = (e_1, a_2)$. Because a_1 is above m_1 the first jump j_1 is from $\hat{L}_1$ to L_1 and the second jump j_2 is from L_1 to $\hat{L}_1$. **Bottom:** A graphical representation of h_2. The initial condition is the point $p = (a_1, a_2)$ and $h_2(p) = (e_1, a_2)$. Because a_1 is below m_1, the first jump j_1 is from $\hat{L}_1$ to R_1 on the LP side and from branch R_2 to $\hat{L}_2$ on the PD side. The second jump j_2 is from R_1 to $\hat{L}_1$ on the LP side and from $\hat{L}_2$ to R_2 on the PD side.

Figure 22.1 illustrates the construction of the map of knees h from the singular system in our example. Because we are considering a network of two neurons, one knee is the Cartesian product of the left branch of the inhibited LP v_1-nullcline ($\hat{L}_1$) with the local maximum of the uninhibited PD v_2-nullcline (M_2), and is thus one-dimensional. This knee can be parameterized by w_1. Two possible phenomena can occur depending on whether we consider a point on the LP inhibited nullcline above or below the local minimum of the uninhibited LP nullcline (m_1). First consider a point p below m_1 as illustrated in the bottom of Figure 22.1. When released from inhibition, the LP coordinate of p jumps to the right branch, causing LP to PD inhibition and an instantaneous lowering of the PD nullcline. This inhibition persists until the LP coordinate reaches the local maximum of the nullcline. If we assume that the PD coordinate is below the local minimum of the uninhibited PD v_2-nullcline, then the PD jumps to the right branch at the conclusion of the LP burst, causing an inhibition to the LP. Thus the LP coordinate jumps to its inhibited left branch. The system then flows until returning to the knee from which the singular orbit originated. Starting with LP coordinate above the minimum of the uninhibited LP v_1-nullcline, as in the top of Figure 22.1, prevents the LP from jumping to its right branch and thus the PD is not inhibited. Thus the map of knees h is a piecewise defined function given by

$$h(w_1) = \begin{cases} h_1(w_1), & if\ w_1 \geq m_1 \\ h_2(w_1), & if\ w_1 \leq m_1 \end{cases} \tag{22.2}$$

where h_1 corresponds to no firing of the LP and h_2 corresponds to a firing of the LP.

With this description of the map h we can begin to explore its geometric and dynamic properties. The first step in this process is to introduce time coordinates to each branch of the slow manifold that plays a role in the definition of h. First consider $\hat{L}_1$. We choose as a reference point the point $j(M_1)$ having the same w_1-coordinate as the maximum of the uninhibited LP slow manifold, M_1. We define the time coordinate τ of a point p with w_1-coordinate ω to be the time to flow from $j(M_1)$ to p. Thus τ is given by the integral

$$\tau = \int_{j(M_1)}^{\omega} \frac{dw}{w_\infty(\hat{L}_1(w)) - w} \tag{22.3}$$

where $v = \hat{L}_1(w)$ is the parameterization of the branch $\hat{L}_1$. On the uninhibited right branch, R_1, we let M_1 be the reference point and define the time coordinate τ of a point p with w_1-coordinate ω to be the time to flow from p to M_1. This is given by

$$\tau = \int_{\omega}^{M_1} \frac{dw}{w_\infty(R_1(w)) - w} \tag{22.4}$$

where $v = R_1(w)$ is the parameterization of the uninhibited right branch of the LP. Each stable branch of the LP and PD slow manifolds is parameterized similarly. Either the maximum of the appropriate uninhibited nullcline or a point having the same w-coordinate is a reference point.

Under most circumstances time coordinates do not generalize to higher dimensional manifolds since two arbitrary points do not, in general, lie on the same trajectory. If, however, the differential equations describing the dynamics on an n-dimensional manifold decouple, as in this example, then given a reference point q, one can define the time coordinates of a point p by applying the ideas described above to each coordinate independently.

The use of time coordinates to parameterize each branch of the slow manifold allows us the define the **compression ratio** of two points p and q across a given jump. Let L and R be a pair of stable branches of a one-dimensional slow manifold and let $J{:}L \mapsto R$ be the function defined by the fast system mapping L to R expressed in time coordinates. The following definition of compression is a modification of a definition due to Somers and Kopell.[7]

Definition 22.1: *The* **compression ratio** $\tilde{C}(p,q)$ *of the function* J *for points* p *and* q *on* L *having time coordinates* τ *and* $\tau + h$ *respectively is*

$$\tilde{C}(p,q) = \frac{J(\tau + h) - J(\tau)}{h}.$$

The **instantaneous compression ratio** $C(p)$ *at* p *is given by*

$$C(p) = \lim_{h\to 0} \frac{J(\tau + h) - J(\tau)}{h} \equiv J'(\tau). \tag{22.5}$$

The compression ratio is simply the ratio of the time distance between the image of p and the image of q under the fast subsystem to the time distance between p and q. This is less than one in absolute value if the time distance between the images is less than the time distance between p and q. Note that because we define time coordinates to agree with direction of flow on each branch of a slow manifold, compression ratios are always positive.

With these tools we can now deduce the qualitative properties of the map of knees. In particular we will show that the derivative of the map of knees is the product of compression ratios and hence is always positive. Denote by H the function h defined in Eq. (22.2) expressed in time coordinates. We begin our computation of H by assuming that the initial point p has LP coordinates above this threshold; thus the LP does not fire in this regime. Denote this component of H by H_1 and write $H_1 = F_2 \circ J_2 \circ F_1 \circ J_1$ where J_1 and J_2 are jumps between branches and F_1 and F_2 are the flows along each branch. Each of these functions are expressed in time coordinates.

We begin by introducing time coordinates on the uninhibited LP left branch L_1. Because there is a critical point E_1 on L_1, we cannot introduce global time coordinates on this branch. Instead we will introduce local coordinates by choosing a pair of reference points. Let both $j(M_1)$ and m_1 be reference points and define the time coordinate of p to be the time to flow from $j(M_1)$ if p is above E_1, or the time to flow from m_1 if p is below E_1. We say that the time coordinate of E_1 is infinite. The first flow F_1 is simply translation by time P_L, where P_L is the time to flow along the uninhibited left branch of the PD. Thus $F_1(\tau) = \tau + P_L$. Similarly, $F_2(\tau) = \tau + P_R$ where P_R is the time to flow along the uninhibited right branch of the PD. It follows immediately that

$$H'_1(\tau) = J'_1(\tau)J'_2(\tau^*) \qquad (22.6)$$

where $\tau^* = J(\tau) + P_L$. Thus the derivative of H_1 is the product of the instantaneous compression ratios associated with each jump.

We note that even though two different reference points are needed on $\hat{L}_1$, $H_1(\tau)$ is continuous and real-valued for all τ in its domain. However, Eq. (22.6) is not valid if p has the same w_1-coordinate as E_1. Let θ be the time coordinate of the point on $\hat{L}_1$ having the same w_1-coordinate as E_1 so that $J_1(\theta) = \infty$. We can make H'_1 continuous at θ by defining

$$H'_1(\theta) = e^{kP_L} \qquad (22.7)$$

where k is the derivative of the singular vector field on L_1 evaluated at E_1. A proof of Eq. (22.7) is given in Reference 4.

We next turn our attention to the component of the map of knees corresponding to LP firing. This function, denoted H_2, has as its domain the set of points on $\hat{L}_1 \times M_2$ with LP coordinate below the minimum of the uninhibited LP v_1-nullcline. As in the previous case, H_2 can be described using the jump-flow-jump-flow paradigm and thus we will again write $H_2 = F_2 \circ J_2 \circ F_1 \circ J_1$.

We claim that in time coordinates the functions F_1 and F_2 are each the identity function. To see this consider the point b_1 on R_1 and b_2 on $\hat{L}_2$ as illustrated in the bottom of Figure 22.1. From this figure we see that $F_1(b_1,b_2) = (c_1,c_2)$ when we express F in a coordinate-free manner. Let τ_1 denote the time coordinate of b_1. The time coordinate of c_2 is the time to flow from b_2 to c_2 which is the time to flow from b_1 to c_1 which is exactly τ_1 since $b_2 = J(M_2)$ and $c_1 = M_1$ are both reference points. Thus in time coordinates we have $F_1(\tau) = \tau$. By similar reasoning it follows that $F_2(\tau) = \tau$.

Let a_1 and c_2 have time coordinates τ and τ^* respectively so that we again have

$$H'_2(\tau) = J'_1(\tau)J'_2(\tau^*) \qquad (22.8)$$

Thus H'_2 is the product of the compression ratios associated with the jumps comprising H_2. Because compression ratios are positive, it follows that H is an increasing function on each of its pieces.

We have shown that H is a real-valued function with a unique jump discontinuity and $H'(\tau) \geq 0$ for all $\tau \neq \theta$. A catalog of possible dynamical behaviors for maps having these properties is given in Reference 4. One possible configuration of H is illustrated in Figure 22.2.

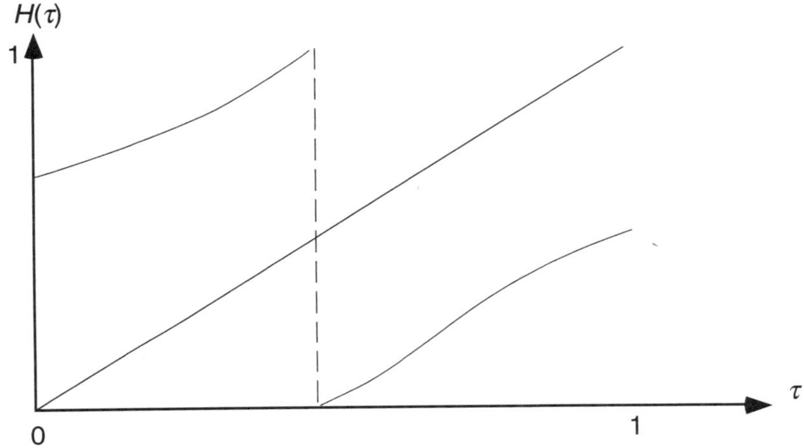

Figure 22.2. The graph of a typical map of knees H after rescaling.

22.3. Biological Implications

In this section we will assume that each periodic orbit of the map H corresponds to a periodic orbit of the model system. Although this is not true for all possible maps H constructed in the manner (see Ref. 1 and 5), it is true for a large enough subset of such maps to make this assumption reasonable. We will further assume that, after a rescaling, H is qualitatively similar to the function illustrated in Figure 22.2, i.e. $H_1(\tau) > \tau$, $H_2(\tau) < \tau$, and $H_1(0) > H_2(1)$.

The dynamics of maps having these geometric properties have been extensively studied by Keener.[2] He has shown that associated with such maps is a well-defined rotation number ρ that measures the average amount of rotation of each iterate when we view H as a map of the circle (identify $\tau = 0$ with $\tau = 1$). If $\rho = m/n$ for m and n positive integers having no common divisors, then H has a periodic orbit of period n. The rotation number ρ depends continuously on parameters with the graph of ρ as a function of a single parameter typically forming a "devil's staircase."

In our example a periodic orbit with $\rho = m/n$ corresponds to a situation where the LP fires $n - m$ times for every n PD bursts. Thus a wide variety of dynamical behavior can occur in such networks. Moreover, the behavior can change dramatically with changes in the model parameters. For example, if two different rotation numbers are observed at two different levels of injected current I, then all rotation numbers between these two values of ρ are observed as I is varied within this range.

In other words, an infinite variety of periodic behaviors occurs in this parameter range.

The results in Reference 4 suggest that this wide variety of possible behaviors is due to the slow recovery of the excitable cell (the LP). If one assumes the recovery rate of this cell to be fast relative to the burst duration of the oscillating cell (the PD), then only two types of behavior can occur: either the LP never fires or the LP fires after every PD burst. Thus the source of dynamical behavior is the assumption of a slow recovery rate.

By contrast, the source of dynamics in slightly more complex models can result from other factors. We have shown that if we assume that the excitable neuron possesses an additional ionic current, known as an I_h current, then the resulting dynamical behavior can be quite different.[3,4] Although the inclusion of this current adds an additional dimension to the problem, techniques similar to those presented here can be used to study the resulting model. In certain parameter ranges, the resulting map of knees exhibits only periodic orbits corresponding to 1 burst of the excitable neuron to every n bursts of the oscillator. This behavior is dependent not on the recovery rate of the excitable neuron, but upon the activation rate of the I_h current as well.

22.4. References

1. C. Bonet, "Singular perturbation of relaxed periodic orbits," *J. Diff. Eqns.* **66** (1987) 301-339.
2. J.P. Keener, "Chaotic behavior in piecewise continuous difference equations," *Trans. of the AMS* **261** (1980) 589-604.
3. T. LoFaro, N. Kopell, E. Marder and S. Hooper, "Subharmonic Coordination in Networks of Neurons with Slow Conductances," *Neural Computation* **6** (1994) 69-84.
4. T. LoFaro and N. Kopell, "Reduction of a network of voltage-gated conductance equations to a one-dimensional map," in preparation (1995).
5. E.F. Mischenko and N. Rosov, *Differential Equations with Small Parameters and Relaxation Oscillations* (Plenum Press, New York, 1980).
6. H. Morris and C. Lecar, "Voltage oscillators in the barnacle giant muscle fiber," *Biophysical J.* **35** (1981) 193-213.
7. D. Somers and N. Kopell, "Rapid synchronization through fast threshold modulation," *Biol. Cyber.* **68** (1993) 393-407.

23. ESTIMATING DOLLAR-VALUE OUTCOMES OF WORKMAN'S COMPENSATION CLAIMS USING RADIAL BASIS FUNCTION NETWORKS

MONTE F. HANCOCK, JR., M.S.
Computer Science Innovations (CSI), Inc., 1235 Evans Road
Melbourne, Florida 32904-2314, USA
E-mail: mhancock@csihq.com

and

Department of Mathematics and Computer Science, Rollins College
Winter Park, Florida, USA

ABSTRACT

This investigation is based upon a data base of outcomes of worker's compensation claims. We consider whether a radial basis function network (RBF) can predict the total dollar value of a claim based upon medical and demographic indicators (MDI's). This work used data from 12,130 workers' compensation claims collected over a period of four years from the state of New Mexico.

Two problems were addressed:

1. How well can the total incurred medical expense for all claims be predicted from available MDI's? For individual claims?
2. How well can the duration of disability be predicted from available MDI's?

The available features intuitively correlated with total medical cost were selected, including type of injury, part of body injured, person's age at time of injury, gender, marital status, etc.. These features were statistically standardized and sorted by correlation with outcome valuation. Principal component analysis was applied (Karhunen-Loeve).

A radial basis function neural network was applied to the feature sets in both supervised and unsupervised training modes.

For sets used in training, individual case valuations could consistently be predicted to within $1000 over 98% of the time. For these sets, it was possible to predict total medical expense for the training sets themselves to within 10%. When applied as blind tests against sets which were NOT part of the training data, the prediction was within 15% on the whole sets. Results on individual cases were very poor: in only 30% of the cases were the predictions for the training sets within $1000 of their actual valuations.

Single-factor analysis suggested that the presence of an attorney strongly decorrelated the data. A simple stratification was performed to remove cases involving attorneys and contested claims, and the procedures above repeated. (Note: the trained machine could correctly predict the involvement of an attorney over 80% of the time.)

Preliminary results based upon the very limited effort applied indicate that the data support population estimates, but not single-point estimates. However, more can be done with the supplied data set, particularly w.r.t. additional stratification and feature enhancement.

23.1. Technical Background / Nomenclature

23.1.1. Classification Problems

Classification is a special case of the general regression problem, for which the range of the regression function is a discrete set. Desired classification decisions are specified at exemplars, and extended throughout the problem domain by tuning the parameters of a decision function. Inputs to the classifier are usually M-dimensional vectors of "features", and the finitely many discrete outputs are the "classes." Given this understanding, many conventional statistical notions (e.g., RMS error, type 1/type 2 errors) apply.

23.1.2. Feature Space, Goal Space, and Parameter Space

The M-dimensional Euclidean space spanned by the vectors of features for a particular classification problem is called the problem's "feature space." Feature space is the domain of the decision function.

The decision function assigns to each feature vector a "class." The set of all classes is "goal space." Goal space is the range of the decision function; it is just a set, and has no topological or algebraic properties.

A decision function is an instantiation of a parameterized decision function model; let this model have L>0 tunable parameters. Each decision function, then, is represented by a point in L-dimensional Euclidean space. This space is called "parameter space." (For a trainable classifier, parameter space will be the domain of an "objective function", which measures the performance of the classifier.)

23.1.3. Trainable Classifiers

If training is understood to be "incremental improvement of performance through experience and self-adjustment", then trainable classifiers can be built.

We describe a typical variant of so-called "supervised "training (examples of known classification available).[1] The process is a closed-loop optimization (see Figure 23.1), during which a fixed collection of feature vectors (the "training set") is repeatedly presented to the classifier. After each cycle of presentations ("epoch"), the overall performance of the classifier is measured via an objective function. The parameters of the decision function are then adjusted in an attempt to increase the objective function's value on the next epoch.

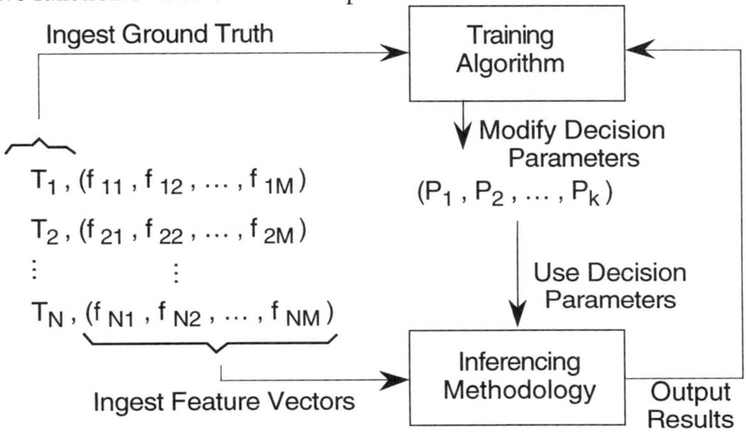

Figure 23.1. Learning by "Feedback and Adaptation."

Training can be regarded, then, as a search of parameter space for global maxima of the objective function with respect to the given training set. Standard optimization techniques may apply (e.g., gradient search, least squares, "filtering" techniques), and emerging techniques are the subject of current research (e.g., back propagation, simulated annealing, genetic algorithms, cascade correlation).[2]

23.2. RBF Networks: Brief Conceptual Tutorial

RBF's attack the regression problem in much the same way "partitions of unity" attack the spectral problem.[3] They operate in the feature space itself, exploiting its geometry to directly model clusters and their boundaries, using many local interpolators of compact support.

RBF's can be regarded as neural networks in the sense that they operate by aggregation of the outputs of many discrete units which are trained rather then programmed. In distinction to most other neural paradigms, however, the elements in an RBF do not communicate with each other.

23.2.1. Stage 1 of the RBF: The Basis Functions

Stage 1 of an RBF's is constructed by positioning at each exemplar in feature space a compactly-supported pseudo-metric. These "basis functions" can be viewed as locally conditioning feature space with a "belief" field, much as an electric charge conditions nearby space with an electric field.

An individual basis function establishes a field of belief that a point in its region of feature space is in the same class as the basis function's exemplar. This belief decreases as we move away from the exemplar, becoming zero at a finite distance. The basis functions are therefore referred to as "radius-limited elements."

To use the basis functions to classify a point in feature space, the outputs of the basis functions in whose support it lies are combined by superposition according to an aggregation rule. This gives a vector of beliefs, component j being the belief that the point is in class j. The largest vector component designates the stage 1 classification. The relative sizes of the beliefs can be used to form a stage 1 classification confidence.

23.2.2. Stage 2 of the RBF: The Perceptron

The stage 1 classification can be used as the RBF output. It is customary, however, to apply a multi-layer perceptron[4] using the original feature vector and its stage 1 belief vector as inputs. The output of the perceptron then becomes the RBF output. (The rationale for using stage 1 as a pre-processor for a perceptron is that the stage 1 procedures can eliminate non-separability, which is problematic for perceptrons.)

23.2.3. The Bayesian Classifier is "Almost" a Stage 1 RBF

The Bayesian classifier is seen to be very similar to a stage 1 radial basis function classifier, with each class represented by a single element located at the class mean, and having local pseudo-metrics given by weighted quadratic exponentials. The only difference is that the exponentials do not have compact support (though in all real implementations, they will have).

The general stage 1 RBF will have many elements representing each class, and possibly different pseudo-metrics. The level-sets of the pseudo-metric give the fundamental shape that is being used to cover clusters in feature space.

23.2.4. Other Interpretations of RBF Classifiers

The stage 1 RBF may also be regarded as a spectral decomposition of the density function for the given classification problem. Properly speaking, of course, this is a spatial rather than spectral decomposition, and the basis functions constitute a frame rather than a basis. This is the sense in which the "partition of unity" analogy with RBF's is instructive.

It is possible at this point to enter a discussion of RBF implementations of fuzzy logic;[5] the connection is obvious, and we forego this.

23.2.5. The Characteristic Strengths of RBF Classifiers

- Unlike most neural paradigms, RBF's radius-limited elements do not extend their interpolation arbitrarily far away from their control points (the exemplars). This gives them good false-positive rejection characteristics by avoiding uncontrolled regression.
- Because the elements do not communicate with each other, it is often possible to add/remove/combine goal classes without retraining existing elements.
- Because the elements have finite support, it is only necessary to fire those in the relevant region of feature space.
- RBF's are insensitive to the number of output classes. (We have successfully built and trained RBF's with over 300 output classes.)
- The decision parameters in RBF's have geometric significance.
- The components of the belief vector can be used to produce "confidence factors."
- The geometric/analytic nature of RBF's is exploitable using many conventional, mature mathematical tools.
- RBF's have been shown to have the theoretical power to handle arbitrary well-posed classification problems; non-linearly separable problems pose no special difficulty.
- Super-fast hardware implementations of RBF's are commercially available (c. 2 microseconds/classification, pipelined). The INTEL Ni1000 chip is the best example.
- RBF's can be designed to produce classifications of hierarchical "granularity." See the discussion of taxonomic decomposition below.

23.2.6. The Characteristic Weaknesses of RBF Classifiers

- Because RBF's model the data from many local approximations rather than from a few population parameters, they typical use more decision parameters than most other techniques (10,000 parameters is not unusual).
- RBF's are easy to "overtrain", that is, they can merely memorize idiosyncrasies of the training set rather than classification knowledge that will generalize.
- Because superposition is a "voting" strategy, RBF's can be sensitive to the presentation cardinalities in the training set.

- Management and use of the large number of RBF parameters can cause software implementations of RBF's to be slow.
- If every vector in an unambiguous training set is used as an exemplar for some basis function, the RBF will generally give a nearly perfect score on that training set; this makes RBF's hard to evaluate without using separate training and evaluation sets.

23.2.7. RBF Training

To train an RBF, we define an objective function, and perform non-linear optimization in parameter space. In general, this includes adjustment of both basis functions locations, and parameters. Geometrically, the RBF level-sets "float around and change shape" in an attempt to best cover clusters and portions of clusters present in the training set.

23.3. RBF Networks: Formal Definition

Mathematical construction of the Stage 1 RBF:

Let Feature space be $\mathbf{R}^\mathbf{M}$.

Let goal space G = {1, 2, ..., K}, so that points in $\mathbf{R}^\mathbf{M}$ fall into one of K classes.

Recall that "exemplars" are feature vectors which represent a particular class. Denote the ith of I exemplars for class *k* by:

$$\vec{F}_{ki} = f(f_{ki1},\ldots,f_{kiM}) \tag{23.1}$$

Define the basis function associated with $\vec{F}_{ki}$ by:

$$R_{ki}(\bar{x}) = 1 - Min\left(1, \sum_{m=1}^{M} P_{kim}(f_{kim} - x_m)^2\right) \tag{23.2}$$

where $\bar{x} = (x_1,\ldots,x_M) \in \mathbf{R}^\mathbf{M}$ and $\vec{P}_{ki} = (P_{ki1},\ldots,P_{kiM})$ is a vector of (tunable) non-negative parameters. (Hence, for this implementation, parameter space is $\mathbf{R}^\mathbf{M}$).

R_{ki} establishes a hyper-elliptical (scalar) field of "belief" in k-membership around the exemplar $\vec{F}_{ki}$. R_{ki} has the following properties:

- the semi-major axes of the field are determined by the parameter vector $\vec{P}_{ki}$
- it is a monotone decreasing function of "elliptical distance" from $\vec{F}_{ki}$
- it attains its maximum of 1 precisely at $\vec{F}_{ki}$
- it is non-negative and has compact support

- it has continuous partials with respect to the parameters P_{kim} for all points having $R_{ki} > 0$.

$R_{ki}(\bar{x})$ is the contribution of exemplar $\bar{F}_{ki}$ to our belief that $\bar{x}$ is in class k.

Typically, there will be multiple exemplars for each class, so the "total belief" that a point $\bar{x}$ is in class k is an aggregation of the beliefs of the class k exemplars:

$$b_k(\bar{x}) = 1 - \prod_{i=1}^{I}\left(1 - R_{ki}(\bar{x})\right) \tag{23.3}$$

This naturally gives rise to a vector field of beliefs $\mathbf{B}:\mathbf{R}^{\mathbf{M}} \to \mathbf{R}^{\mathbf{K}}$ defined by:

$$\bar{B}(\bar{x}) = \left(b_1(\bar{x}),\ldots,b_k(\bar{x})\right) \tag{23.4}$$

$\bar{B}(\bar{x})$ can be interpreted as a joint-membership function, akin to a k-ary probability density.

$\bar{B}$ is the radial basis function constructed from the exemplars. It is trained by optimizing $\bar{P}_{ki}$.

To use $\bar{B}$ to classify points in feature space, select the index of the largest component of $\bar{B}(\bar{x})$. The b_k's can be used to build confidence factors.

For points far away from all exemplars ("uncontrolled" regions of feature space), $\bar{B}(\bar{x}) = \bar{0}$. The RBF refuses to make "wild guesses."

23.4. The Data

This investigation is based upon 12,130 workman's compensation claim records ('DCI records'). These records are in an 85 field format. They are sampled from claim forms filed in the state of New Mexico between 1988 and 1992. Supporting documentation included a data concordance, coding tables, and a description of the sampling methodology.

23.5. The Problem

Several problems were addressed:

1. Is it possible to predict from DCI phenomenology the total incurred medical expense? That is, can we correctly predict the value of DCI field 60 from the other fields?
2. Is it possible to predict from DCI phenomenology the duration of disability? That is, can we predict the difference of DCI fields 38 and 37 from the other fields?

3. Is it possible to predict from DCI phenomenology which claims will result in litigation/adjudication? That is, can we correctly predict the values of DCI fields 70 and 71 from the other fields?

23.5.1. Preliminary Analysis of the Data

Preliminary analysis was performed to determine general population parameters. The distribution of outcomes (in terms of medical dollars) is heavily skewed to the low end: over 99% of the claims have valuations under $100k.

Single-factor Bayesian analysis, scientific visualization techniques, and covariance measures show low cross-correlation of most factors.

Many vacant fields were found in the set supplied. In order to insure that any results obtained could be applied in practice, we restricted our attention to only those field present in virtually all records.

It was determined that too few DCI records had field 38 present (1452 records out of 12,130) to address problem 2 above.

Preliminary cluster analysis indicated that the supplied estimates of future medical costs were very poor; that is, for DCI records representing open cases, DCI field 60 should be regarded as corrupt for the purposes of our study. Further, our system should aim to improve on current estimation techniques rather than replicate their shortcomings. In the sequel, we restricted our attention to closed cases only (DCI field 34 = 4).

23.5.2. Feature Extraction

The features satisfying the above conditions which are intuitively correlated with total medical cost were selected. Some of these were synthesized from multiple DCI fields:

1. Type of Injury
2. Part of Body
3. Person's age at time of injury
4. Gender
5. Marital Status
6. Age of policy at time of injury
7. Employment status at time of injury
8. Retained attorney?
9. Claim ever contested by carrier?
10. Type of employment
11. Traumatic, occupational, or cumulative injury?
12. pre-injury weekly wage

These features were statistically standardized and sorted by correlation with outcome valuation. Principal component analysis was applied.

The data set was divided into four smaller sets: A, B, C, and D. Each of these smaller sets held approximately 1100 normalized case records.

23.5.3. Training Methods

Our taxonomic radial basis function neural network was applied to the feature sets A and C. This was done in both a supervised and unsupervised training mode. For sets A and C (those used in training), individual case valuations could consistently be predicted to within $1000 over 98% of the time.

For both sets A and C, it was possible to predict total medical expense for the training sets themselves to within 10%. When applied as blind tests against sets B and D (which were NOT part of the training data), the prediction of total population claim value was within 15% on the whole sets. Results on individual cases were very poor: in only 30% of the cases were the predictions for the training sets within $1000 of their actual valuations.

Single-factor analysis had suggested that the presence of an attorney strongly decorrelated the data. A simple stratification was performed to remove cases involving attorneys and contested claims, and the procedures above repeated. (Note: the trained machine could correctly predict the involvement of an attorney over 80% of the time.)

After stratification, the blind test set results improved to estimation of total aggregate reserving dollars to within 0.5% on set B, and 7% on set D. However, individual case estimates were still poor.

23.5.4. Preliminary Conclusions

Preliminary results based upon the very limited effort applied are not promising. More can be done with the supplied data set, particularly in additional stratification and feature enhancement, but indications are that the data provided do not support single-point outcome prediction.

23.5.5. The Need for Additional Data

All appearances are that further progress will be constrained by the limitations of the supplied data set. Holes in the supplied data set forced consideration of only a few of the 85 collected features. Aggregate results were consistently much better than individual results. The data set had to be subdivided to provide for blind tests. These facts, coupled with the high resolution ($1000 bins) desired on the output side indicate that the supplied data set does not adequately cover the universe of discourse.

23.6. Biography

Monte F. Hancock, Jr., MS, is Chief Scientist and Director of Research and Development at CSI, and also serves on the Adjunct Facility of Rollins College, in the Departments of Mathematics and Computer Science. He is listed in the current edition of "Who's Who in the South and Southwest."

Computer Science Innovations, Inc. was founded in 1983 in Palm Bay, Florida and is currently active in a wide variety of markets. From a beginning based on the design and development of custom, state-of-the-art Information Management Systems for the Command, Control, Communications and Intelligence (C^3I) marketplace, CSI now participates in both DoD and commercial markets. CSI's main business is solving our customers hardest problems using innovative solutions and the latest in technology.

CSI is headquartered in Melbourne, Florida and has branch offices in the Baltimore-Washington area and Central America.

Tel: (407) 676-2923   Fax: (407) 676-2355

23.7. References

Hecht-Nielsen's book is undoubtedly the best general reference available on neural networks. The author knows of no definitive general reference on radial basis functions. The RBF paradigm is a little over 10 years old.

1. R. Hecht-Nielsen, *Neurocomputing* (Addison-Wesley, 1990), p. 7.
2. B. Kosko, *Neural Networks for Signal Processing* (Prentice Hall, 1992).
3. J. Dugundji, *Topology* (Allyn and Bacon, 1973), pp. 169-171.
4. E. Rich and K. Knight, *Artificial Intelligence* (McGraw-Hill, 1991), pp. 492-500.
5. B. Kosko, *Neural Networks and Fuzzy Systems* (Prentice Hall, 1992).

24. A NOVEL APPROACH TO MODELING AND DIAGNOSING THE CARDIOVASCULAR SYSTEM

LARS J. KANGAS, PAUL E. KELLER, SHERIF HASHEM
Pacific Northwest National Laboratory†*, P.O. Box 999, K1-87*
Richland, Washington 99352, USA
E-mail: lj_kangas@pnl.gov, pe_keller@pnl.gov

RICHARD T. KOUZES
Department of Physics, West Virginia University, P.O. Box 6216, 302 Stewart Hall
Morgantown, West Virginia 26505, USA
E-mail: rkouzes@wvnvm.wvnet.edu

and

PAUL A. ALLEN, M.D
Life Link, Inc., 949 Stevens Drive
Richland, Washington 99352, USA

ABSTRACT

In this paper, a novel approach to modeling and diagnosing the cardiovascular system is introduced. A model exhibits a subset of the dynamics of the cardiovascular behavior of an individual by using a recurrent artificial neural network. Potentially, a model will be incorporated into a cardiovascular diagnostic system.

This approach is unique in that each cardiovascular model is developed from physiological measurements of an individual. Any differences between the modeled variables and the variables of an individual at a given time are used for diagnosis. This approach also exploits sensor fusion to optimize the utilization of biomedical sensors. The advantage of sensor fusion has been demonstrated in applications including control and diagnostics of mechanical and chemical processes.

24.1. Introduction

A model of an individual's cardiovascular system must mimic the relationship among physiological variables (i.e., heart rate, systolic and diastolic blood pressures, and breathing rate) at different physical activity levels. If a model is adapted to an individual, then it becomes a model of the physical condition of that individual. A model for a healthy individual can be compared to the actual measure-

†This work was supported by the Laboratory Directed Research and Development Program at Pacific Northwest National Laboratory (PNNL). PNNL is a multiprogram national laboratory operated by Battelle Memorial Institute for the U.S. Department of Energy under Contract DE-AC06-76RLO 1830.

ments of that individual at a later time. Any differences can be exploited to evaluate and diagnose medical conditions that affect the cardiovascular system of that individual. When used in clinical exercise testing (e.g., graded exercise tests), these cardiovascular models will increase the sensitivity of correctly diagnosing several medical conditions such as those listed in Table 24.1. These models will also increase the sensitivity of detecting or excluding several other conditions that cannot be uniquely diagnosed in an exercise test alone such as those listed in Table 24.2 (Jones 1988, Lamb 1984, Pollock 1990).

Table 24.1: Conditions detectable with exercise testing.

myocardial ischemia
peripheral vascular disease
exercise-induced asthma
vasoregulatory asthenia
unfitness
vasoregulatory asthenia
psychogenic dyspnea
muscle phosphorylase deficiency

Table 24.2: Conditions not directly detectable with exercise testing alone.

chronic bronchitis
pulmonary emphysema
pulmonary infiltration, alveolitis, and fibrosis
pulmonary thromboelism and hypertension
congenital cardiac abnormalities
cardiac valvular obstruction or incompetence
primary myocardial disease
generalized neuromuscular disorders

A cardiovascular model can be incorporated into an automatic, continuous diagnostic system carried on a person. Physiological variables received from noninvasive biomedical sensors can be compared with the modeled variables in real-time. This real-time diagnosis of an individual's general health increases the possibility of early detection of undesired medical conditions and reduces the response time of medical help for people working in hazardous and dangerous environments, (e.g., soldiers and law enforcement officers). A real-time diagnostic system also enables continuous monitoring of people with medical conditions in nursing homes and in home-care situations. Reduction of the response time for medical help is critical in minimizing medical complications and the loss of life.

Initially, we expect that employees working in hazardous environments would be monitored for early diagnoses of a degradation in health. The working environment and other causes may contribute to this degradation and make an employee unsuitable for certain work. For example, the described system could aid fire districts in determining the health effects from smoke inhalation on individual firemen. The system would determine whether firemen have recovered sufficiently from the last inhalations of smoke to be allowed to enter smoke-filled environments again.

The cardiovascular model is being developed with artificial neural network (ANN) technology. ANNs have been applied to modeling complex process dynamics for the manufacturing and chemical industries. We hypothesize that cardiovascular systems exhibit similar dynamics and can be modeled with ANNs. Additionally, ANN technology could be used to build the diagnostic system since they have already been successfully applied to a variety of medical diagnostic systems (Baxt 1991, Dorffner 1994, Jones 1990, Kennedy 1991, Mango 1994, Rosenberg 1994, Suzuki 1993).

24.2. ANN Based Cardiovascular Modeling

One approach to cardiovascular modeling is to build a model representative of a group of individuals with similar characteristics (i.e., sex, age, physical condition, medical condition, etc.). However, cardiovascular behavior is unique to each individual (Vander 1990), thus a generic cardiovascular model used in a medical diagnostic system would not be as sensitive as a system based on a model that is adapted to the patient being diagnosed. To develop these models without a cardiovascular expert, the modeling must be based on an adaptive technology that can be automated. The ANN technology fits this category.

The ANN technology was selected for the cardiovascular modeling because of its many capabilities including sensor fusion, which is the combining of values from several different sensors. Sensor fusion enables the ANNs to learn complex relationships among the individual sensor values, which would otherwise be lost if the values were individually analyzed. In medical modeling and diagnosis, this implies that even though each sensor in a set may be sensitive only to a specific physiological variable, ANNs are capable of detecting complex medical conditions by fusing the data from the individual biomedical sensors.

Recurrent ANNs were selected for the cardiovascular modeling application to capture the temporal information in physiological variables. These variables are time-series data from which both the absolute values and the rates of change need to be modeled. Recurrent ANNs recycle a small portion of information from time t-1 at time t. Indirectly, decreasing portions of information from time t-2, t-3, t-4, etc. are also captured, thus enabling recurrent ANNs to model the temporal dynamics in data. Figure 24.1 illustrates a prototype tool that generates an ANN model of the cardiovascular system from physiological variables received from biomedical sensors attached to an individual.

During the adaptation phase, the training algorithm receives physiological data from an individual via biomedical sensors and automatically develops the ANN-based cardiovascular model. After development, the model can generate the appropriate physiological responses for simulations with varying levels of physical activity. Figure 24.2 shows how the variables modeled with the ANN compare with the physiological variables generated with a nonadaptive cardiovascular model. This second model has been used for creating data with sufficient complexity for the development of the modeling tool.

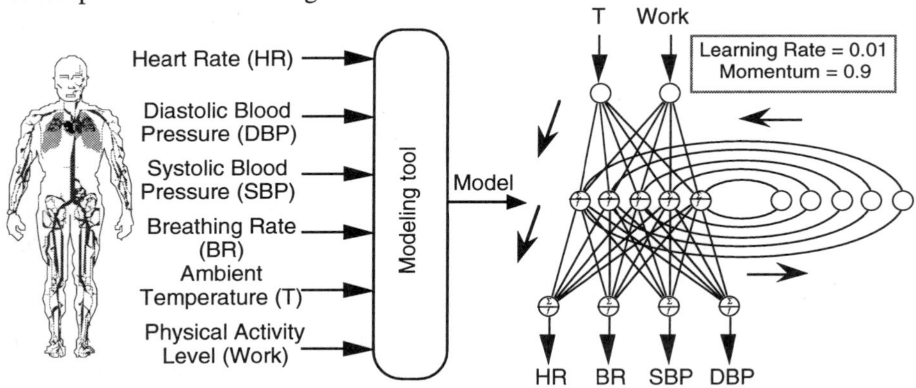

Figure 24.1. On the left, this figure illustrates a modeling tool that takes a sequence of physiological variables from biomedical sensors and learns the temporal dynamics of these variables to produce an ANN-based cardiovascular model. On the right, this figure illustrates the configuration of the ANN produced by the modeling tool. The ANN has two inputs, four outputs, and five hidden processing elements. The ANN takes the ambient temperature and the physical activity as input. The four outputs, heart rate, breathing rate, systolic blood pressure, and diastolic blood pressure, are clamped to the "actual" values during the training phase. For the initial cardiovascular model prototypes, the "actual" values are generated by a nonadaptive cardiovascular model. During the modeling phase, the temperature and the work are input to the ANN, and the values at the outputs are taken as the modeled variables. The feedback links going through the five processing elements on the right side of the ANN enable it to capture temporal information in the data.

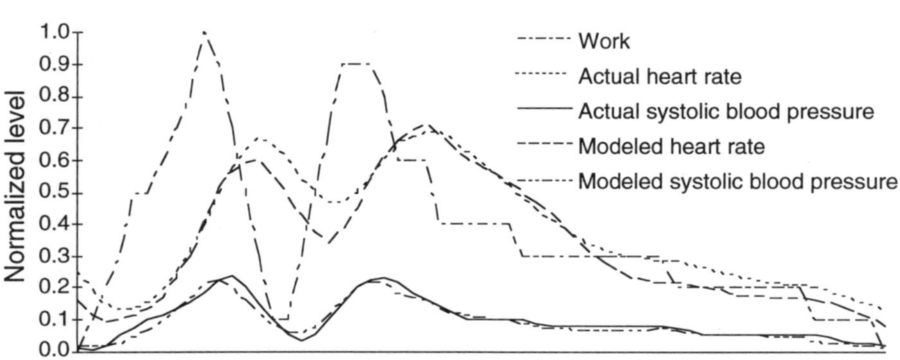

Figure 24.2. This graph depicts the "actual" and modeled heart rate, and the "actual" and modeled systolic blood pressure for varying physical activity levels. The "actual" variables in this graph are generated with a nonadaptive cardiovascular model. The vertical axis corresponds to the normalized magnitude of these variables (normalized to one). The variables for systolic blood pressure and breathing rate are excluded from this figure for clarity. The effects of varying ambient temperature has not yet been explored in this research.

24.3. Model Based Cardiovascular Diagnostics

It is envisioned that cardiovascular models will be incorporated in both clinical diagnostic systems for graded exercise tests and cardiovascular stress tests, and in an automatic, continuous diagnostic system carried on a person.

The methodology for using models as a basis for diagnosis is often referred to as "model-based reasoning." Diagnostic systems that use model-based reasoning compare actual data to modeled data and exploit the differences for diagnosis. Two prerequisites for this methodology to be successful are that the models are authentic to the systems being diagnosed and that the differences between the modeled data and the actual data are known for diagnostic conditions.

Conventional modeling techniques tend to build generic models with possibly a few free variables that fit the model to an instance of a system. For example, a respiratory system model-based on differential equations may have a few free variables adjusted to an individual's sex, age, and weight (Tehrani 1993). An ANN-based model is potentially a superior model because almost all of its free variables are adjustable to behave as a specific instance of a system.

Conventional diagnostic techniques most often require that the differences between the modeled and actual data are known to the person developing the diagnostic system. These techniques are handicapped by both the ability of the person to understand the diagnostic differences in the data and by the applicability of those differences to the modeling technique. An ANN-based diagnostic system is potentially superior because it does not require a priori knowledge of the diagnostic differences in the data, although it should be recognized that some knowledge aids the development.

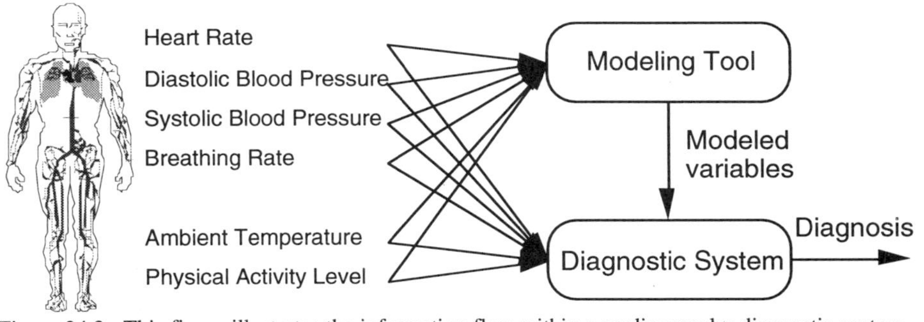

Figure 24.3. This figure illustrates the information flow within a cardiovascular diagnostic system that uses model-based reasoning to produce a diagnosis of health by comparing a model of an individual to the individual's current condition.

A diagnostic system based on a model uses an individual's normal-condition cardiovascular behavior as a reference. Any variation from that behavior indicates a change from the normal condition. An ANN-based diagnostic system is trained to recognize the effects of certain medical and physical changes on the monitored variables. For example, a blood loss results in a decrease in blood pressure and an increase in heart rate relative to the normal values for that individual. Figure 24.3 illustrates a diagnostic system and the information flow in model-based reasoning. The modeling tool receives the physiological variables from an individual via biomedical sensors. The diagnostic system receives the same variables from both the biosensors and the model. These two sets of variables are "compared" for diagnosis.

24.4. Discussion

This paper introduced a prototype diagnostic tool that models a subset of an individual's cardiovascular system and uses model-based reasoning to determine the individual's health. The modeling tool learns the dynamics of the relationship between physiological measurements for an individual observed at different physical activity levels. Because a model adapts to an individual, it duplicates the physical condition of that individual. As such, it can be employed in "what-if" medical scenarios to evaluate and diagnose medical and physical changes.

A tool of this type is envisioned to serve in two broad areas. First, it would serve in personal health diagnostic systems for continuous diagnosis of health and for periodic clinical tests: graded exercise tests and cardiovascular stress tests. For example, a real-time diagnostic system using these cardiovascular models may be used to monitor the health of workers in hazardous environments or to monitor and control administration of medication for hospital patients. Second, it can function as a simulator for biological systems used in education and research related to the human physiology and as a controller for medical mannequins.

In future work, this research will include the modeling of additional physiological variables, specifically variables describing pulmonary gas exchange: oxygen uptake (V_{O_2}), and the concentrations of carbon dioxide (CO_2) and nitrogen (N_2). A complete physiological exercise test should also include multichannel electrocardiography (ECG). After completion of the cardiovascular modeling tool, a model-based reasoning diagnostic system will be developed with ANNs.

Information on ANN developments at Pacific Northwest National Laboratory is available in the World Wide Web (WWW) pages of the Environmental Molecular Sciences Laboratory. This information is accessible through WWW clients such as NCSA Mosaic. The uniform resource locator for this site is

http://www.emsl.pnl.gov:2080/docs/cie/neural/.

24.5. References

W.G. Baxt, "Use of an artificial neural network for data analysis in clinical decision-making: The diagnosis of acute coronary occlusion," *Neural Computation* **2** (1991) 480-489.

B. Blumenfeld, "A Connectionist Approach to the Processing of Time Dependent Medical Parameters," *Proceeding of the 1990 International Joint Conference on Neural Networks*, (Washington, DC, 1990), Vol. 2, pp. 575-578.

G. Dorffner, E. Leitgeb, and H. Koller, "Toward Improving Exercise ECG for Detecting Ischemic Heart Disease with Recurrent and Feedforward Neural Nets," *Proceedings of the IEEE Workshop on Neural Networks in Signal Processing*, (Ermioni, Greece, 1994).

D. Jones, "Neural Networks for Medical Diagnosis," *Handbook of Neural Computing Applications*, (Academic Press, 1990), pp. 309-318.

N. Jones, *Clinical Exercise Testing*. 3nd edition (W.B. Saunders Company, Philadelpia, 1988).

R.L. Kennedy, Robert F. Harrison. S.J. Marshall, and C.A. Hardisty, "Analysis of clinical and electrocardiographic data from patients with acute chest pain using a neurocomputer," *Q J Med.* **80** (1991) 788-789.

D.R. Lamb, *Physiology of Exercise: Responses and Adaptations*, 2nd edition. (MacMillan Publishing Company, New York, 1984).

L.J. Mango, "Computer-assisted cervical cancer screening using neural networks," *Cancer Letters* **77** (1994) 155-162.

M.L. Pollock and J.H. Wilmore, *Exercise in Health and Disease: Evaluation and Prescription for Prevention and Rehabilitation*, 2nd edition (W.B. Saunders Company, Philadelpia, 1990).

C. Rosenberg, J. Erel, and H. Atlan, "A Neural Network that Learns to Interpret Myocardial Planar Thallium Scintigrams," *Neural Computation* **5(3)** (1993).

Y. Suzuki, Y. Abe, and K. Ono, "Self-organizing QRS Wave Recognition System in ECG using ART2," *Proceedings of the World Congress on Neural Networks*, (Portland, OR, 11-15 July 1993), Vol. 4, pp. 39-42.

F.T. Tehrani. "Mathematical Analysis and Computer Simulation of the Respiratory System in the Newborn Infant," *IEEE Transactions on Biomedical Engineering* **40** (1993) 475-481.

A.J. Vander, J.H. Sherman, and D.S. Luciano, *Human Physiology: The Mechanisms of Body Function* (McGraw-Hill Publishing Company, New York, 1990).